D0907337

The ULTIMATE Career Guide for Nurses

DATE DUE

The WHMCLE Career Guide for Nursing

The ULTIMATE
Career Guide for Nurses

Practical Advice for Thriving at Every Stage of Your Career

Donna Wilk Cardillo, RN, MA, CSP

LIBRARY
MILWAUKEE AREA
TECHNICAL COLLEGE
NORTH CAMPUS
5555 West Highland Road
Mequon, Wisconsin 53092

ANA
AMERICAN NURSES ASSOCIATION

610.K9
C267
2018

Library of Congress Cataloging-in-Publication Data available upon request

The American Nurses Association (ANA) is the only full-service
professional organization representing the interests of the nation's 4 million
registered nurses through its constituent/state nurses associations and
its organizational affiliates. The ANA advances the nursing profession
by fostering high standards of nursing practice, promoting the rights of
nurses in the workplace, projecting a positive and realistic view of nursing,
and lobbying the Congress and regulatory agencies on healthcare issues
affecting nurses and the public.

ISBN print   978-1-947800-12-0
ISBN ePDF   978-1-947800-13-7
ISBN ePub   978-1-947800-20-5
ISBN mobi   978-1-947800-14-4

© 2018 American Nurses Association
8515 Georgia Ave., Suite 400
Silver Spring, MD 20910

All rights reserved.

First printing, August 2018

To the memory of Richard N. Bolles, author of What Color is Your Parachute?, *who wrote the foreword to the first edition of this book. His words and his work continue to inspire me.*

Brief Contents

Contents

Acknowledgments

Thank you to Erin Walpole and Eric Wurzbacher and all of the great editorial and design staff at the American Nurses Association; Marcia Blackwell for her editorial and research assistance; all the experts who contributed to the original version of this book as well as this updated edition; the thousands of nurses I have interviewed, talked with, and worked with over the years who shared their stories, their challenges and their triumphs; my amazing family including Helen, David, Justyna, Sebastian, Junior, Pia, Barbara, Barry, Anna, Ed, Nancy, Mimi, Andrew, Matthew, Pam, Paul, Lily, Max, Jasper, Rose, Eugene, and Linda; and my amazing husband Joe, who is my constant support and inspiration, advisor, proof reader, editor, and comic relief.

Introduction

Florence Nightingale is quoted as saying, "Nursing should not be a sacrifice, but one of the highest delights in life." And it is for that reason that I wrote this book: to support every nurse in creating the most fulfilling, meaningful, and joyful career possible. In fact, there has never been a more exciting time to be a nurse. With each passing day we are creating and working in more expanded roles, extending both our reach and our impact. And while our challenges may seem bigger, so too are our opportunities.

So much has changed in nursing, health care, and the world at large since I published the first edition of *The ULTIMATE Career Guide for Nurses* in 2008. While hospitals have been the foundation of our health care delivery system for decades, care is shifting out of the acute care arena into alternate inpatient settings, ambulatory settings, the home, and the community. Likewise, wellness promotion and prevention have taken center stage. Nurses are starting businesses in record numbers, and more and more nurses hold top leadership roles in health care facilities, government, and private health care businesses.

As more and more is demanded of us, and as we choose to elevate and expand our role, we must hold ourselves to a higher standard of evidence-based practice, educational preparation, and emotional intelligence. Clinical skills and credentials are no longer enough to move our individual careers and nursing's agenda forward. Much of what worked for us in the past won't work in the future. Knowledge and information, not to mention the demographics and healthcare needs of the public, are constantly changing.

What hasn't changed is the fact that nursing continues to be the most diverse profession on the planet. Whether going from home to home in rural areas or serving as the CEO of a large health care system, nurses are leading the way by providing high-quality, cost-effective, compassionate care. We touch lives and we change lives.

Richard Bolles, author of the classic book *What Color is Your Parachute?*, had been gracious enough to write the foreword for the first edition of *The ULTIMATE Career Guide for Nurses*. Unfortunately for the world, he has since passed away. But in that foreword he recalls how, as a former hospital chaplain, one nurse said to him, "Home. Hospital. Supermarket. Church. Week after week. That is all there is to my life." This describes how some nurses fall into a rut, become stagnant, and lose touch with the bigger picture. Then one day they find themselves woefully out of date and often out of a job with few prospects for good employment.

Today's nurse must be proactive in their career: always learning, moving forward, acquiring new skills, staying abreast of industry changes, willing to change their mind and perspective on key issues in practice and culture, making a commitment to self-care, finding balance in personal and professional spheres, and always being proud of who they are and what they do. That is what *The ULTIMATE Career Guide for Nurses* is all about.

Florence Nightingale was tough and outspoken, an excellent communicator who was persuasive and effective in making her point. She was well educated, socially savvy, politically active, and an adept networker. Fiercely passionate about her work, she used the power of her connections to move nursing forward. She didn't blame anyone for the social barriers she encountered or try to figure out why they existed. She just broke through them and kept on going. She had vision, determination, confidence, and a strong sense of self. Today's nurse must embody these traits, not only to keep the profession strong but to remain joyful, passionate, relevant, and resilient.

Here's to your success, longevity, and sheer joy in nursing. Look out world, here come the nurses!

Chapter 1

This Profession We Call Nursing

In spite of all the changes in health care today, nursing still offers rich and diverse opportunities. For those willing to leave old stereotypes behind, to step outside their comfort zone, and to avail themselves of all that this glorious profession has to offer, the challenges, rewards, and means for self-actualization and fulfillment are great.

Many nurses believe that nursing is not a job, but a career. What's the difference? A job is simply something you show up for every day. You put in your hours, go home, and then repeat the cycle the next day. Very little ever changes and your work is routine and mundane. You operate on autopilot, resist change, and work to collect a paycheck. You stay in one place until you get bored, get fired, or retire. Some people stay with a job even though they're bored or burnt out because they fear making changes or believe they have no options. They get into a rut and can't seem to get themselves out.

On the other hand, a career is something you plan for and work at. It constantly evolves and expands whether you work in one place or move around during your professional life. A career is like a living, breathing organism that changes and grows over time. It needs continuous nourishment through new experiences, education, risk taking, and challenges. And while a career requires a solid base, it is pliable enough to adapt to an ever-changing environment. Career management involves feeding, weeding, and constantly reshaping your career landscape. It is a perpetual cycle of renewal and growth, a process of stretching yourself and always moving in a positive forward direction. Managing your career keeps your professional life fresh and active, alive and well. Learning to effectively manage your career will lead to a happier, more fulfilling, and more rewarding career. It's the antidote to stagnation and will increase your longevity in this profession.

Managing your career also puts you in the driver's seat. Nurses have more control over their workplace and professional lives than they realize. They also have more opportunities than they are aware of and possess more skills and abilities than most give themselves credit for, even right out of nursing school. And while nursing skills are acquired in school, how to manage and nurture a career is often something you must learn on your own.

The components of an effective career management plan include:

- Knowing your industry and keeping abreast of changes,
- Knowing yourself through self-assessment and self-awareness,
- Developing goals and creating a plan of action,
- Taking calculated risks in your career for advancement and growth,
- Trying new things and stretching yourself,
- Being proactive rather than passive,
- Getting into a cycle of continuous formal and informal learning,
- Becoming proficient at self-marketing,
- Developing professional networks,
- Maintaining career mobility, and
- Achieving a healthy balance between professional and personal lives.

Unfortunately, many nurses don't understand the concept of career management. It is not something you do only when looking for a job. Rather, career management is an ongoing activity designed to get the most out of your current job and your career in the long run.

I once attended a convention where I was representing Nurse.com at its exhibit booth. I was giving out copies of their annual career management guide. When offered a complimentary copy, many nurses declined, saying, "No thanks, I'm not looking to change jobs," or "I don't need that; I'm happy where I am." Another began to shake her head back and forth and said, "Oh, no. I've got my heels dug in where I am and will be there until I retire." I found these reactions interesting and amusing as clearly these nurses equated anything to do with career management with changing jobs. The guide contained much more than how to find a job. For example, it had articles about public speaking, self-care for nurses, email etiquette, time management, and how to make the most of meetings. It also addressed usual clinical and nontraditional specialties and even issues such as investing and how to get out of debt. All of these things are elements of an effective career management plan.

The reaction I received at the convention is not uncommon. Many nurses believe that as long as they are employed, all is well. Employment becomes their security blanket, conveying a false sense of stability. They become comfortable and insulated and don't feel the need to stay fully connected to the world around them. It's amazing how many nurses are certain they will never need to look for another job. However, jobs don't last forever, and nurses may not want to or be able to stay in their present jobs in the future. Let's face it, job security is an illusion. Whether we are experiencing a nursing shortage or surplus, no one is immune to lay-offs, reengineering, mergers, buyouts, and other workplace changes. Here are a few other situations to consider: What if you became disabled or developed a back or shoulder injury? What if you decided to go back to school and needed a flexible schedule, or simply wanted a different lifestyle at some point? Plus, everyone is living and working longer these days so the likelihood of spending our entire career in one specialty, role, and place of employment is unlikely. These are realities to think about. Here's another scenario: Things may be just fine where you are now until a new manager or administrator is hired and everything changes.

I once spoke with a long-time operating room (OR) nurse. In the course of conversation, I asked her if she had thought about what she would do if she ever decided to leave the OR. She quickly responded, "Oh, that will never happen. I love what I do, and people will always need surgery." I reminded her that while people will always need some type of surgery in our career-lifetime, more and more surgery is being done on an outpatient basis, new technology is enabling less-invasive procedures, and fewer people need certain types of surgery because of more sophisticated diagnostics. One nurse told me that a multihospital system recently purchased her hospital and all of the employees had to reapply for their own jobs.

Nurses with the mindset of the OR nurse I spoke to will be unprepared for the inevitable shifts in a workplace.

One thing is guaranteed—your job is going to change, whether you stay where you are or not.

Whether you're happy in your current position, looking to make a change, exploring your options for the future, or just wanting to take your career to the next level, career management should be a part of everything you do. If you are not actively managing your career, then you can't very well complain about your circumstances.

What Is a Nurse?

When asked what we do, many nurses lapse into industry jargon about performing assessments, administering medications, monitoring health status, and other similar things. But nursing is less about the tasks we perform and more about a knowledge-based practice that plays a key role in every aspect of health care.

What is a nurse? A nurse is a combination of education, experiences, skills, abilities, and the capacity to care and to give. We as nurses are not defined by where we work or whether or not we wear a uniform or scrubs to work. It is about who we are. Nurses are vital at the bedside, but we are just as vital in every other aspect of the health care arena. We have been making a difference in many ways and places since the beginning of our profession.

What do nurses do? We promote health and wellness. We facilitate entry into this life and departure from it. We touch lives and we save lives. We bring light into dark places. Nurses are scientists, teachers, nurturers, and healers. The world has always needed a lot of healing—of the mind, body, and spirit. We are caregivers, patient advocates, researchers, educators, lobbyists, change agents, managers, administrators, counselors, and business owners. And sometimes we are simply another human being sharing in the experience of life and death.

Being a nurse is not something you turn on and off. Nurses are never off duty. If someone in our family or in our circle of friends gets sick or needs health care advice, we are on. We are vigilant to the health needs of the world. Even today as a nurse–entrepreneur traveling the world, speaking, writing, and coaching, I am a health advisor and educator, telephone triage nurse, bereavement counselor, first-aid provider, home care nurse, and care planner and coordinator for my extended family and friends. Once a nurse, always a nurse.

Nurses do many different things in many different places. One of the great things about this profession is an endless opportunity for each nurse to meet their interests, special skills, scheduling needs, physical ability, and location. There is never a reason to be bored. However, the general public, and even some nurses, have a deeply entrenched view that nurses work almost exclusively at the bedside in a traditional role. When you tell people you're a nurse, often the first thing they ask is, "What hospital do you work in?" The moment I stepped out of the hospital years ago into a nontraditional nursing role, people would ask me why I left nursing. Some nurses even still think that those who work in nontraditional roles are not "real" nurses, a view that frames us in a limited capacity. It boxes us in and confines us to one specific role and work setting. This perception views nurses as one-dimensional. Then when we try to get out into the world to be visible, vocal, and taken seriously, people want to know what we're doing outside of the hospital. That same mentality is what makes people wonder what a woman is doing outside of the kitchen.

Some people fear that nurses would be lured away from bedside nursing if they knew about non–direct care options, as if keeping nurses in the dark is the way to keep them at the bedside. On the contrary, many nurses truly love bedside nursing and wouldn't do anything else. In fact, some nurses who left the workforce or had taken on administrative or nontraditional roles are now looking to return to bedside nursing. For them, bedside care is nursing at its best because that's where the action is and their hearts are.

Some nurses do need or want a less physically demanding environment, have specific scheduling needs, or simply wish to put their knowledge and skills to work in a different way than the bedside. Other nurses got into the profession with a specific goal of working in public health, developmental disability nursing, wellness promotion or education, addiction services, or other nonhospital, nonbedside roles. I suggest that we need to embrace an expanded view of who we are and what we do as a profession. It's time to celebrate the role diversity within nursing. It's time to revel in our accomplishments and contributions, whether at the bedside or in the boardroom, whether doing research or calibrating IV pumps, whether dressed in pumps and pearls or scrubs and clogs. We are all in the same profession trying to make an impact, trying to make positive changes, and doing our part. Although we are all different people, we share one heart, one soul, and one voice as nurses.

Am I still a nurse today, as a writer, speaker, and entrepreneur? You'd better believe it. I am just as much a nurse standing in front of an audience in a business suit, or sitting at my computer in jeans as I was when I wore a white uniform and cap and worked in the emergency department (ED). I am still a teacher, nurturer, and healer in everything I do. I just do it in a different way. My philosophy, values, and mission haven't changed. I have no doubt that I am still contributing to the greater good of health care. I am a nurse first and a business owner second. Once a nurse, always a nurse.

Changing Times

As the world around us changes, health care and nursing change, too. For starters, the population is rapidly aging. We're all living longer and even though we're healthier and more active than previous generations as we age, the older we get, the more health care services we need.

Because of continuously escalating costs in health care, we are constantly looking for innovative ways and places to deliver good quality, cost-effective health care. Hospital care is expensive and is an often less than ideal setting for meeting the health care needs of many populations. And with an epidemic of chronic illness in the United States and increasing need for ambulatory care services instead of acute care services, we are seeing a gradual decrease in hospital admissions (with subsequent hospital closings across the country) along with a gradual increase in outpatient services. All this has shifted care from the traditional hospital to the home, community, and alternate care settings, including subacute care, rehabilitation, and long-term care. Patients who do come into the hospital are likely sicker and stay for a shorter period of time than in the past.

Technology is now an integral part of health care to test, diagnose, and, in some cases, even treat and monitor patients from remote locations. Computers also allow us to keep better records and manage the flow of information. They are great tools for education and research. We continue to see advances in medical and nursing practice and research. Significant progress has been made in the areas of transplantation, genetic engineering, and the manufacture of artificial body parts and human organs, such as skin and corneas, which are now being grown in labs. We have better diagnostics and treatment modalities, less invasive procedures, and more effective drugs.

The traditional health care community, including health insurance and managed care companies, has shifted its past focus on acute illness to staying well and managing chronic illness. Western medicine has largely embraced holistic practices and philosophies that treat the whole person, rather than solely a specific disease process. We're now focusing as much on promoting lifestyle changes and managing stress as we are on more traditional interventions. Many nurses have incorporated mindfulness or present moment awareness training into their practices, including teaching yoga and meditation. Our society is looking for more natural, more effective, and more interdisciplinary solutions for staying well and healing. Perhaps we're getting tired of being poked, prodded, and medicated, too.

We've also seen a resurgence of spirituality and a reemerging sense of community in this century. However, this century's society is increasingly violent, plagued not only by global terrorism but by local issues of domestic violence, child and elder abuse, and sexual abuse and assault. More of these events are reported these days, and more victims are coming forward for treatment and justice, which is a step in the right direction.

These industrial and societal changes have prompted new, exciting specialties in nursing and have expanded some others. Some examples follow in the paragraphs below.

Clinical nurse leaders (CNLs) take clinical practice to the next level without becoming advanced practice nurses. According to the Clinical Nurse Leader Association (CNLA) web site, CNLs are master's-prepared advanced generalists who work at point of service and focus on coordinating, facilitating, and overseeing evidence-based practice, safety, quality, risk reduction, and cost containment (CNLA 2017).

Nursing informatics specialists manage implementation and maintenance of electronic medical records and other uses of information technology (IT) in the delivery of health care. They facilitate interface between clinicians and IT in many ways including education, research, and practice, such as supporting virtual services in inpatient and outpatient settings.

Care managers (not to be confused with case managers) work one-on-one with people with chronic illnesses or disabilities and their loved ones in various settings. They function as liaisons with insurance companies and health care providers, help manage medications, create plans of care, research treatment options, and more. They also are known as geriatric care managers, nurse concierges, professional patient advocates, and nurse navigators.

Holistic nurses promote health, wellness, and healing from a whole-person perspective. They assess, teach, coach, and counsel consumers and staff and in some cases incorporate modalities and practices such as Reiki, meditation, yoga, and essential oils. These nurses may work in any practice setting incorporating a holistic approach to care.

Nurse case managers focus on care coordination, financial management, and resource utilization to yield cost-effective outcomes that are patient-centric, safe, and provided in the least restrictive setting, according to *Nursing Case Management: Review and Resource Manual* (Leonard & Miller 2012, 21).

Wellness coaches work with individuals and groups to set and achieve health goals. This service is being offered by hospitals, managed care companies, medical homes, nurse entrepreneurs, private health promotion companies, and nurse-led clinics.

Home health nurses provide a broad range of services including care coordination, care management, disease management (management of an individual chronic illness), hospice and palliative care, mother–baby services, wellness and prevention, education, coaching, and more—all key components of the new health care paradigm.

These are just a few examples of new and expanding specialties in nursing in response to changing times. The nursing profession is constantly changing, evolving, and adapting as things around us change and as we continue to expand our own vision of who we are, what we are capable of doing, and how we fit into the system.

Changing Workforce

Several decades ago, the profile of the typical nursing student was a young woman right out of high school. Most attended hospital-based training programs, and few went on to higher education. All that has changed.

With an increasingly complex work environment, the ever-expanding role of the nurse, and significant research linking better patient outcomes to baccalaureate and higher education for nurses, a BSN degree has become standard in many settings. And while associate's degree nursing programs are still active, most graduates of these programs recognize that higher education must be in their future.

Although men and minorities still represent a small percentage of overall RNs, the data show that those numbers are increasing.

More and more people are coming into nursing as a second, third, or fourth career. Therefore, many students and newly licensed nurses are older and bring diverse work experience with them into nursing. Many of these "multicareerists" come to the profession with degrees in other disciplines.

Some nurses enter the nursing profession with the specific goal of becoming a nurse practitioner (NP), certified registered nurse anesthetist (CRNA), certified nurse midwife (CNM), or even nursing administrator after obtaining prerequisite experience.

All of the above elements will only serve to strengthen nursing in the future. We have to be open to new ways of thinking and doing things. There would be no progress without that. Nothing stays the same. We must move forward.

Why are people coming into nursing today? Most men and women come to nursing for the same altruistic reasons that nurses of past generations did. Some multicareerists have become disillusioned with the corporate world or blue-collar job they came from and want to do something more meaningful with their lives and careers. Also, the spotlight on the helping professions as a result of terrorism and other tragic events at home and abroad has brought to light the important role that nurses play in health care. And, of course, a good job market with ever-expanding opportunities, including advanced practice roles, doesn't hurt either.

One Nurse's Journey

I can't recall the exact moment I decided to become a nurse, but I remember developing a love affair with the profession early on. I always loved science, and I couldn't think of any area more interesting than human science. While in high school, I worked as a candy striper in a hospital and felt energized by the fast-paced human drama that surrounded me. I remember the sense of awe I experienced entering the inner sanctum of the intensive care unit (ICU) with dinner trays. I recall the excitement and joy of walking past the nursery window and seeing all that new life squirming and fussing. I remember the emotion in the voices of family members and friends who would call for information about the status of their loved ones. I recall how my heart would beat faster when an ambulance sped down the street and into the ED driveway. I can still see all the important-looking people walking around with a sense of purpose on their faces. And most of all, I remember the patients.

I used to love to watch old movies about hospitals, and I fell in love with the image of the nurse: the starched white uniform, the cap, the sensible lace-up oxford shoes. A good friend gave me my first pair of Clinic shoes as a high school graduation gift, and she couldn't have given me anything better. I should have had those shoes bronzed when I finished with them, they were so symbolic to me. Little did I know at the time all the miles and all the places those shoes, and subsequent pairs, would take me in this glorious profession.

On my journey, I began to learn that people who are not nurses often do not understand what the profession is all about and what we get out of it. They often say, "I could never do what you do," or "I don't know how you do it." Outsiders see only the challenges and hardships, such as dealing with human pain and suffering, working long hours, and dealing with difficult people. What nonnurses could not possibly see or know is the overwhelming sense of contributing to the greater good, of making a difference in the lives of others, of being there for people during their darkest and most vulnerable hours, and of impacting the health and wellness of the population. It's difficult to explain the feeling we get when someone looks into our eyes and says, even without words, "Thank you. I'm so glad you're here." Or when someone who wasn't expected to live or walk again somehow recovers and goes home largely as a result of good nursing care and support. It is the reward of caregiving.

I also found that a common misunderstanding people who aren't nurses have is that nurses are somehow a rung or two below physicians in the health care chain. Every nurse has been asked at one time or another in their career, "Gee, you're so intelligent. Why didn't you become a doctor?" implying that intelligent people become doctors and not-so-intelligent people become nurses. Because the profession has always been predominantly female, I sometimes hear people say that women did not have many career choices in the past and that's why many chose nursing when they were younger. What they fail to realize is that many of us knew we had options and believed we could be whatever we wanted to be. And still we made a deliberate and enlightened choice to go into nursing. I was born to be a nurse. There is nothing else that I would do, even today. Nursing has been the ride of my life.

> ## "WHY DIDN'T YOU BECOME A DOCTOR?"
> Jackie says, "The best response I ever heard was, 'Why on earth would I want to be an MD? I have the best possible position [as a nurse] for getting to know and helping people over the long term.'"

When I started out more than 30 years ago, like many nurses I had only images of nurses at the bedside. I presumed that was what I would always do. A modern-day Florence Nightingale, that was me. During nursing school, I had an opportunity to work part-time as an electrocardiograph (ECG) technician. That experience introduced me to the ED. I spent a great deal of time there and was intrigued by the fast pace, the diversity of cases, and the precision with which everyone seemed to work. It was almost like watching a ballet with beautifully choreographed movements, crescendos, and diminuendos. Later in school I worked in the ED as a nurse's aide and grew to love it.

I had some great psychiatric nursing instructors in school who were so enthusiastic about the specialty that I too developed a keen interest in it. So, while a student, I also worked in a county psychiatric hospital, which was home to many chronically mentally ill men and women. Many of the patients I encountered there had been abandoned long ago by family members or had simply outlived their relatives and had nowhere else to go. This environment was very different from the ED and offered very unique challenges. In the ED, patients came and went quickly. We treated and released people or stabilized them before moving them out to another department. In the county psychiatric facility, I had the opportunity to develop long-standing relationships with patients and learn about their families, histories, and backgrounds. I was already discovering the diversity that the profession had to offer me. Needless to say, both environments were eye-opening for me.

Upon graduation, there were no openings in the ED where I worked as a student, so I initially worked in another facility that offered extensive psychiatric services. As a new nurse, I was ready to take on some challenges. I chose to work in a locked ward for male patients. This unit served as an admission ward for those with addictive disorders, those with court-ordered 72-hour admissions, county prisoners who required psychiatric evaluation, and any other acute psychiatric admissions. Here I began to better understand the complexities of the human mind. My patients had significant substance abuse problems, were accused of violent crimes, came from abusive and dysfunctional homes, suffered from severe depression, were homeless, or had various acute and chronic mental illnesses. Some nurses have an aversion to psychiatric nursing, but I found it to be one of the most fascinating and challenging specialties.

Still, my heart was in the ED. So when I heard about an opening in my old department, I grabbed the opportunity. The ED exposed me to the full spectrum of the human experience on a moment-to-moment basis. Even though I was working in a small community hospital, I saw my share of trauma and other medical and surgical emergencies. I also saw many patients with run-of-the-mill medical complaints and chronic illness, those who didn't have a family physician or insurance coverage, and those who just thought it was easier to come to the ED than get an appointment. I even assisted with the occasional birth of an overly eager baby in a car in the ED driveway.

WHY CHOOSE NURSING?

Barb recollects choosing nursing as a profession:

"I remember my aunt, who was an author, telling me I could 'do better than that' and be a doctor or a writer, as I so love to write. She would often say, 'Why be just a nurse? You're wasting yourself in such a lowly profession.'

"But you know, when she was dying of breast cancer almost three years ago, I stayed at her house with her (she lived alone) for her last two weeks. I felt honored to be able to be there as her favorite niece...and, as her nurse. The night before she died, she said: 'What would I do without you? Thank God you're a nurse.' This was the last thing she said to me. I still get a heart tug every time I remember this."

In the ED, I developed a true appreciation for the sacredness and fragility of human life. I loved the ED because I was exposed to many specialties: cardiac, obstetrics (OB), pediatrics, orthopedics, neurology, and psychiatry. Because of my mental health background and their psychiatric nursing phobia, my coworkers assigned the psychiatric patients to me. My ED also doubled as the outpatient department for the hospital. That meant we ran outpatient clinics for all specialties and performed procedures like colonoscopies, blood transfusions, and minor surgery. We were also a poison control center, and ran public screening programs for diabetes, mouth cancer, eye health, and other services. There was very little I wasn't exposed to in that ED, one way or another.

At the time, I presumed I would always work as an ED nurse—that's who I was, that's what I did. But then I got married and bought a house far from where I was working. I had to leave my beloved ED to look for employment in a new location. I thought I would just find another job in an ED in my new neck of the woods because that's who I was, and that's what I did. I began to scan the classified ads, but the ED positions advertised were almost all for the evening or night shift. That was not conducive to my life-style as a newlywed.

Expanding My Horizons

When I couldn't find a day job in an ED, I began to explore other options. I noticed an ad for a part-time job in a medical weight control center. I needed a full-time job, but I was intrigued by the position and wanted to learn more. Besides, I figured maybe I'd have access to some of their secrets and actually lose a few pounds if I worked there! I picked up the phone and made an appointment for an interview. After the usual questions and answers about the job, the nurse conducting the interview said, "Would you by any chance be interested in a full-time position?" I agreed enthusiastically. She continued, "It just so happens we have a head nurse position open in a center in your area. Would you consider that?" "Yes," I replied, while having no idea what I was in for next. With that, she escorted me down the hall to meet with the president of the company. I was totally unprepared for this. I thought I would breeze in, get a little information, and go on my merry way. I hadn't even dressed that well because I had interviewed more out of curiosity than a belief that I would receive a job offer of any kind.

I was now in the inner sanctum of the executive offices of this multi-location New Jersey company, dressed way too casually, and feeling scared and overwhelmed. I was introduced to the company president, and he began asking me real interview questions, such as, "What are your goals?" I don't believe I had any goals back then. I was in a state of panic because as a nurse, I had never had an actual interview in my life. Years ago, interviews for nurses consisted of one question: "When can you start?" Yet as a nurse, I was accustomed to thinking on my feet. And like many nurses, I was more intelligent than I gave myself credit for at the time. I answered his questions as best I could and apparently did OK because at the end of the interview he said, "Well, congratulations. You have the job!"

Bewildered, I asked, "Well, excuse me, but which job do I have?" I was so confused at that point.

The company president responded, "The head nurse position!" I thought it was pretty good that I applied for a part-time staff position and left with a full-time management position.

Was this a fluke? Not at all. It has happened to many nurses before and after me. In fact, this sort of thing happens all the time when you get out there and interview. I had applied to what is known as an "open job," one that is publicly advertised and usually has many competing applicants. I left with what is known as a "hidden job," an opening that exists in a company that is not publicly advertised. Hidden jobs account for the majority of available positions out there. I learned a valuable lesson: an interview is always an opportunity.

Looking back, this was a perfect transitional position for me. I was expected to work in my white uniform and cap (traditional nurses' garb at the time) and would be drawing blood and taking ECGs, so I still felt like a "real nurse." I learned a lot about nutrition and the mechanics of weight loss and gain, including physiological and psychological factors. I counseled and taught patients and offered lots of support. I was also learning a little about the business side of health care. And for those of you who are wondering, I did lose some weight while I worked there, but I gained it all back after I changed jobs!

Just a Nurse?

About 10 months into my new job, the company president asked to have lunch with me. I was a little nervous, but knew that I was thought well of in the company and felt confident that I was doing a good job. Shortly into lunch he blurted out, "The manager in your center is being transferred to another location, and I'd like you to take over managing that center." I was dumbstruck. If I had been swallowing food at that moment, I would have needed the Heimlich maneuver. I broke out into a cold sweat and began to stutter and sputter and flail my arms as I proclaimed in a high-pitched voice, "I can't do that. I'm just a nurse!" To further my point I added, "I don't know anything about human resources, advertising, selling, or management. Thanks, but no thanks." I presumed I had effectively put an end to his absurd notion.

With a slight smile on his face, the businessman sat there considering my reaction and what I had just said. I couldn't imagine what he found amusing. Finally, he said very emphatically, "I understand your reluctance, but I think you can do the job. I *want* you to take it." He wasn't giving me a choice. I had once heard that if you are offered a promotion on the job and you don't accept it, you might not have much of a future with that company. For that reason alone, I reluctantly accepted the position of center manager.

> Being a nurse is not something you turn on and off.

Once the decision was made, I experienced panic I had never felt before. Maybe it wasn't as bad as when I had to give my first injection to a person rather than a navel orange, or the time I found myself alone in a psychiatric ward with a six-foot five-inch 350-pound psychotic man who had just thrown a chair through a window, or the time.... OK, OK, I think I made my point. Let's just say that I spent a miserable, sleepless weekend wondering what I had gotten myself into. I lost respect for this man. How could he put someone like me in charge of one of his business ventures? What was he thinking? I figured it would probably take me 3–6 months to completely run the business into the ground. It would just be a matter of time before I was pounding the pavement again, looking for work. No one was more convinced than I that I would fail miserably in this new position.

As if that wasn't enough, I now had to wear street clothes to work, and I didn't have any. I had a typical nurse's wardrobe: white uniforms and casual clothes. I had no idea what to wear to work unless it was white and sold in a uniform store.

The big day finally arrived. I threw together an outfit, took a few deep breaths, and told myself I'd been in tougher spots than this. For instance, there was that time in the ED when.... You get my gist.

An amazing thing happened once I started in my new position. Slowly but surely, like everything else in life, I began to learn what I needed to know to manage that center. I learned by asking questions, by doing, by observing experienced people, and sometimes just by figuring things out on my own with trial and error, which nurses are very good at. In fact, I learned it all so well that 8 months later, the owner of the company asked me to open and manage a second center for him. By now, I had the management thing down pat, so I said, "No problem." I had certainly come a long way, and I began to fully appreciate all the skills and attributes I possessed as a nurse.

Let me assure you that in comparison to what we have learned in nursing school and during our practice, acquiring business skills is easy. However, because it is different from what we are accustomed to, we might assume we can't do it. But how often have you encountered a new procedure or piece of equipment or been pulled to work in an unfamiliar unit? You always adapt, learn what you need to, and find a way to get the job done. It's the same thing elsewhere. But take nurses out of the hospital, and they often forget what they are capable of. Nurses are smart. I know this because we need to be to get through nursing school, pass a rigorous state licensing exam, and do what we do every day. We are also multitalented and versatile, qualities in ourselves that we often miss.

As you can imagine, managing two centers was a 24-hours-a-day, 7-days-a-week responsibility. After working at this company for several years, my personal circumstances changed. I was now looking for something that was strictly 9 AM to 5 PM, Monday through Friday, and low stress. The ideal job for some, right? I even wanted something close to home so I could walk to work if needed. Again, I began combing the classified ads looking for something different and, hopefully, interesting. I saw an ad for a part-time staff position in an office that did medical exams for insurance companies. They were not even looking for a nurse, but the work sounded intriguing and the office was a few blocks from where I lived. I needed a full-time job, but decided to go on the interview anyway. During the interview, the woman asked, "Would you by any chance be interested in a full-time position?" I gleefully replied, "Yes. Actually, I need a full-time job." She responded, "It just so happens that our office manager is getting married and moving out of state. Would you be interested in that position?" I could hardly believe this was happening for the second time. Now that I had some management experience under my belt, I eagerly told her I was interested.

With that, she brought me in to meet the franchise owner. At least I had dressed better this time. I'd learned my lesson the first time around. At the end of the interview, I was offered the position of office manager. The salary was much lower than what I had been making in the weight control center, but I weighed sanity and a regular schedule above that. I accepted the position and figured I'd find a way to make ends meet.

Once again, I applied to an open job and left with a hidden job. In both positions, I had applied for a part-time staff position and left the interview with a full-time management position. Is this because I was lucky and just in the right place at the right time? I don't believe so. You have to be open to all possibilities as they present themselves. Sometimes you have to take a chance and go on an interview, even if you're not sure what's involved. An advertisement never tells you everything there is to know about the position, employer, or other opportunities that may be waiting in the wings. Once again, this experience illustrates how *an interview is always an opportunity.*

In this new position, I had to take incoming phone calls from insurance agents about life insurance policies they sold. I determined what the medical requirements of their company were for issuing the policy and assigned the case to one of our medical field examiners. These examiners were nurses, chiropractors, emergency medical technicians, and other health care workers. They went to the person's home or office, completed a medical history, and checked vital signs. I then reviewed these histories for clarity, completeness, and accuracy. Keep in mind that my employer had not used nurses in my position before. He used to train laypeople to do these reviews. However, as a nurse, I picked up inconsistencies or things that needed clarification on these exams that only a person with a health care background could detect. He was impressed with my knowledge and was getting compliments from the insurance agents on the accuracy and completeness of the exams. I got my first raise shortly thereafter.

While working for this company, revolutionary changes were taking place in health care reimbursement. The diagnostic related groups (DRG) system was introduced in the United States, and it would eventually replace the old itemized billing method. This complex and then-controversial system required categorizing inpatients based on their admitting diagnosis along with other medical conditions and treatment factors. Code numbers were assigned to elements in the patient's medical record. This categorization and coding would determine how much reimbursement the hospital would get for that patient's care.

The parent company of the franchise I was working for decided to expand their business and start doing hospital bill auditing and DRG coding verification. Because I was one of the few nurses employed by this national company, they asked if they could train me in the DRG system and have me go out on a few calls to hospitals on a trial basis. Of course, always being open to learning something new, I said yes. To be honest, it was also an excuse for me to get away from my usual routine in the office. Little did I know at that time how valuable this experience would be.

All of this ultimately led me to one of the best jobs I had in health care—the director of DRG services in a community hospital. This was during a time when hospitals were hiring DRG coordinators to manage the rapidly changing regulatory and reimbursement issues coming down from insurance companies, the government, and other agencies. My new employer was looking for a nurse who had familiarity with reimbursement issues. The job was tailor-made for me. Additionally, I'd be back working in a hospital, on my home turf so to speak, which made me happy.

What made it even more exciting was that this was a brand new position. I would be responsible for building the department from scratch. I had my own office and was considered part of the management team reporting directly to the hospital administration, not nursing administration. That was a big change for me—and an eye-opening one. I had officially become a member of what other nurses have dubbed the "pearls and pumps" group, those who wear business suits to work.

Keep in mind that I got the previous job, which led me to this challenging, prestigious position, by applying for a part-time staff position where they weren't even looking for a nurse and were not paying a great starting salary. You never know where the road will take you when you allow yourself to venture outside your comfort zone into the world.

After that, I worked for a managed care company as the health services manager and later worked for an education company that provided review courses to help new graduates pass their state licensing exams. With each new position, I learned something new about myself and about the health care industry. I'm still learning as I continue on my journey.

Nursing is a very specific career choice—one filled with challenges, rewards, and endless pathways forward. Nurses are versatile and multitalented. We are vital at the bedside, but we are just as vital in every aspect of the health care arena. And just as things around us are constantly changing, so must each of us grow and evolve and keep moving forward to fully take advantage of all that nursing has to offer and to reach our full potential as human beings and as professionals. So let's discuss how you can maximize your opportunities and find long-term happiness and fulfillment in this profession we call nursing.

Chapter 2

Everyday Career Management

Now that we've established that every nurse should be engaged in career management on an ongoing basis, let's discuss the basics. Obviously, you need to complete specific tasks if you're looking for another job, want to change specialties, or have your sights set on moving up the corporate ladder. But all nurses should maintain basic aspects of their career regardless of their current situation. Let's talk about building a foundation first and move forward from there.

Join a Professional Association

Joining and becoming active in professional associations is a key element of professional success. These organizations hold many opportunities for personal and professional development and growth. They are an essential part of ongoing career management. You cannot develop a career in a vacuum, and that's exactly what you're trying to do if you don't join and get active in your professional associations.

It is through our professional associations that we create community in nursing. Without being connected to that local, national, and international community, you may survive but you will not likely thrive in nursing.

Professional associations provide a forum for disseminating information, providing education, and lending support. They function as a collective voice for people who have common interests and concerns. At the same time, they allow the exchange of ideas among members with diverse opinions. If you think everyone in an association is of one mind, you haven't been out to any meetings lately!

Professional associations are invaluable resources for every nurse from student to retiree. While some well-meaning people encourage nurses to join their professional associations merely out of support for that organization, that is not the best reason to join. You should join because of the personal and professional benefits and opportunities. Here are some examples of what's in it for you.

Membership Has Its Rewards

By joining a professional organization, you become part of a group that forges immediate bonds with other members. If you call or email other members or run into them somewhere, camaraderie arises just from the affiliation, even if you don't otherwise know one another. You have a sense of belonging and being part of a greater whole. And professional associations are some of the best places to find role models, coaches, and mentors. There are other rewards of membership:

- You start getting related print and electronic publications—local, statewide, and maybe even national ones. This is one of the best ways to stay on the cutting edge of the most current knowledge and information about your profession and specialty. You'll find out about upcoming educational and networking events, learn about legislative issues that may affect your practice and license, and be in the know on other key industry topics.

- You have a resource whenever you need information, referrals, or answers to questions about your profession. Whether your concerns are clinical, ethical, legal, or simply career-related, you can just pick up the phone or send an email for a timely expert response or at least a good referral.

- You become entitled to benefits and features reserved for members only. For example, some organizations offer exclusive career services or specialty committees and caucuses for advanced practice, nursing informatics, and other special interests. Many associations offer scholarships, support groups, and in some cases, financial support during illness or hard times. You might get access to special areas of the association's web site, such as online advice, continuing education (CE) offerings, private chat forums, social media groups, and specialty-specific information such as salary surveys, demographics, and industry trends.

- You'll receive member discounts to conventions, CE and special programs, and other products and services.

- You gain a competitive edge that nonmembers may not have. For one thing, the affiliation looks good on your résumé. Memberships in professional associations show that you are an involved and informed professional. This appearance can make a difference when changing jobs, seeking a promotion or transfer, being nominated for an award, qualifying for a clinical ladder, or being considered for other positions and opportunities both inside and outside of your place of employment.

- You have access to powerful and influential people. Because most industry leaders belong to their professional associations, you'll get to rub elbows with the best and the brightest in your profession. That alone can be inspiring. And when people outside the organization are looking for nurses to interview, spotlight, appoint to a government committee or task force, or speak at an event, they often turn to professional associations first.

Go to a Meeting

By attending the meetings of your professional associations, you'll have an opportunity to meet nurses from other facilities, specialties, and roles. These gatherings are great opportunities to mix and mingle. They provide a forum for sharing information and ideas and finding out what's happening in other places of employment. Not only can you pick up some ideas to bring back to your own department, but you gain perspective on the work world beyond your own job. You can't get a sense of whether things at your workplace are typical or not if you don't know what's happening in other workplaces.

Other benefits of attendance are listed below:

- You have an outlet to let off some steam. Many of us don't take time to socialize with our colleagues and have fun. We isolate ourselves and foster a sense of being alone. Even if things are less than ideal where you work, it's comforting to know that others are in the same boat. You can commiserate and even laugh about your common situation, taking comfort in knowing that others share your experience. And attending professional association meetings can be a good excuse to get out of the house for a while.

- You'll always learn something new, either from a CE presenter, an exhibitor, or another meeting participant. And you'll meet some of the most interesting people you'll ever encounter.

Find a Committee and Join

By participating in a committee, you'll gain maximum benefit from your membership. You get out of any organization what you put into it. Join a committee that interests you or one where you can develop your special talents. Want to learn more about legislative issues, lobbying, or policy development? Join the political action committee (PAC). Interested in teaching and speaking? Join the education committee. Have an inclination toward writing or marketing? Get on the newsletter or public relations committee. Love event planning? Volunteer to work on the annual convention or a fundraising project. There are two other benefits derived from committee work:

- You gain more visibility within the organization when you become active. People get to know you better and vice versa. And for those of you who are shy about meeting new people, this is a great way to overcome your shyness.
- As a committee member, you'll have the opportunity to hone your communication, negotiation, and conflict management skills. You may even learn about finances, marketing, and budgeting. You'll gain experience working with a group and develop your leadership skills.

Don't Miss Live Events

By attending annual conventions and special programs, you become enlightened, energized, and empowered. Conventions, legislative days, and special educational programs are great ways to stay connected to peers and industry leaders on a broader scale. There are always local and statewide events to attend, and if you haven't been out to a national convention or meeting in a while, you don't know what you're missing. The experience of meeting colleagues from all over the country face-to-face is unparalleled—you find out just how similar nurses from different regions are. A few added advantages of attending events are listed below:

- You'll gain access to industry leaders, such as editors, authors, administrators, educators, researchers, clinicians, and association leaders. I almost always attend my state association of the American Nurses Association (ANA) convention because anybody who's anybody in the nursing profession in my home state is usually there. There's nothing like meeting notables in person, having an opportunity to shake their hands and get face time with them.
- You'll have the opportunity to speak with exhibitors from other places of employment, schools of higher education, professional

associations, and businesses that offer products and services for nurses and other health care professionals. It's a great way to get a lot of information in one place and stay abreast of what's happening in your industry and specialty.

- You'll have an opportunity to attend keynote presentations, educational sessions and workshops, and pick up some CE credits while doing it. I guarantee you'll come back home with ideas, information, renewed enthusiasm, and new friends.

Go to an Awards Ceremony

These events are a celebration of nursing. Awards dinners and galas highlight all the incredible things nurses do every day to make a difference and all the good that is possible to achieve. And with all the negative images and messages about nursing out there, attending awards ceremonies is one way to reinforce the power and passion of nursing. Regardless of what you do in nursing, seeing your colleagues honored gives you a sense of pride, inspiring and renewing your faith in the profession. Such events remind you what nursing is all about and why you got into the profession in the first place, while listening to the wonderful accomplishments of others can give you something to work toward.

Seek an Elected Position

By running for office, you are forced to step outside of your comfort zone and stretch yourself. The experience builds character, whether you are elected or not. It's also a great opportunity for visibility within the organization.

If you're successful, your position can provide one more reason to interact with other members. One shy colleague of mine once told me that she felt much more comfortable introducing herself to others in the organization because of her elected position. For example, she would introduce herself by saying, "Hi. I'm Janet Rivers, the vice president of programming." She felt that her position gave her the status and confidence to initiate conversations that would have been difficult for her otherwise.

An added benefit of elected office in a professional organization is the impression it can make on current and prospective employers. It demonstrates that you have leadership skills, that you hold the respect of your peers, and that you are a person who can get things done. It looks good on your résumé, too. Holding office in a professional association carries more weight and influence than members believe at first.

Usual Objections to Joining Professional Associations

Some nurses have created an extensive litany of unworthy excuses for nonparticipation in their professional organization. Seasoned by time, but unable to stand up to the scrutiny of a moment, they include the following:

I don't have time to get out to meetings. No one has much free time these days, but we all make time for those things that are important to us. The education, the support, the camaraderie, and the "fun factor" discovered at meetings will be beneficial to you and your career. You'll also develop your social skills. Even if you can't get out to meetings regularly, you'll still have all the other privileges and benefits of membership, plus you can participate in online forums and groups.

The dues are too expensive. Cost is relative to value. I guarantee you'll get more than your money's worth if you avail yourself of all the association has to offer. Besides, your dues are probably tax-deductible if you itemize, so talk with your tax preparer about that and other deductions related to professional association membership and participation. Some associations have special rates or payment plans for students, new graduates, retirees, disabled members, and unemployed members. Some employers may even reimburse you for your professional memberships. It doesn't hurt to ask.

I won't get anything out of it. In short, active membership is the best way to stay on the forefront of knowledge and information about your specialty and profession. It also provides a forum for sharing ideas and information, and is a wonderful way to support and celebrate the nursing profession. You can learn and develop your special interests and talents. It's a great way to meet nurses from other facilities and specialties, gain access to industry leaders, and find role models and mentors. In the end, membership energizes you and gives you a competitive edge.

If you don't belong to professional associations, you become an observer with an obstructed view of your profession as it grows, rather than an active participant. By becoming involved, you become part of the solution, rather than part of the problem.

You can find a comprehensive list of professional associations in the Resources section at the back of this book.

If you're still not ready to join for some reason, go to a local meeting as a guest. I don't know of any professional association that doesn't welcome guests to their meetings. This way, you can check out the programs and the people first before making a decision to join. Attend with a friend or coworker or go solo. Similarly, you can attend conferences and conventions as a nonmember. It's also OK to join now and ease your way in slowly. Even if you only get out to a few meetings the first year, that's progress!

It's important to belong to both the American Nurses Association (ANA) and state ANA association as well as relevant specialty associations. You'll get something different from each one for a well-rounded perspective and experience in the profession. Some nurses only belong to their specialty association and become isolated from the larger nursing community. Stay connected, involved, and informed on every level.

Robin says, "I belong to the Academy of Medical-Surgical Nurses (AMSN). This organization has helped me develop as a professional and nurse leader to heights I never imagined possible. Becoming certified in your area of expertise also demonstrates your commitment to the profession and the welfare of your patients."

Work on Your Education

Ongoing education is a necessary part of career and professional development. So much changes in our daily lives and nursing practice that you have to incorporate learning into your everyday routine. Education is not just about career advancement—it's about staying involved and active. If you're not learning, you're stagnating.

Education can be formal or informal. Let's discuss the formal bit first. Many nurses cringe at the thought of returning to school in any capacity. But unless you already have an advanced degree, formal education should be in your plans. If you want to be taken seriously in nursing, you need essential educational credentials. More important, formal education will enrich your life in ways you can't imagine.

A bachelor's degree has become a minimum standard for any professional today. For those who attended a diploma or associate's degree program, start making plans to return to school for a bachelor's degree in nursing. Don't just think about it, do it. And once you have a bachelor's degree, start thinking about graduate school. Some programs will allow you to work on your bachelor's and master's degrees simultaneously.

I often hear nurses say, "I'm going to retire in a few years," or, "I don't want to get into management, so why should I go back to school?" Formal education will support your career in many direct and indirect ways. However, the personal benefits far outweigh any potential career benefits. Education is a gift you give yourself. It keeps your mind active and young and makes you feel alive. Education helps you to see life in an expanded way with a better understanding of yourself and the world around you. It allows you to participate in a grander way and stay relevant. *Go back to school for yourself first and your career second.* Even if they are planning to retire soon or stay in their current positions, many nurses end up shifting their plans unexpectedly, by choice or circumstance. You never know when and how a degree will come in handy. It's something that will always be a part of you.

Usual Objections to More Schooling

When enrolling in school, don't think about how old you'll be when you graduate. That's sure to sabotage your plans. Just get started, keep moving forward, and eventually you'll get to the end. Additionally you'll want to avoid the following objections and self-imposed barriers to continuing your formal education.

I'm not smart enough. That's the way a lot of us feel, but every nurse is intelligent. How do I know that? Any licensed nurse has gotten through nursing school and passed a rigorous licensing exam. Plus, nurses handle complex situations every day. If you made it this far as a nurse, you can definitely go the distance in higher education. It may not be easy, but you'll amaze yourself when you stretch your mental capacity and see just how much you are capable of learning and mastering. Formal education, once completed, will validate your intelligence.

I don't have the time. Most of us have little free time, but we do have the ability to set aside time for things that are important to us. You may have to give up some volunteer work, delegate household chores, or pay someone to mow your grass or run some errands. There are all sorts of creative solutions to time challenges. Keep in mind that it's a temporary situation.

I don't have the money. Few of us have much disposable income, but more money is available for education than most people realize, and with a little time and effort you can finance all or part of your schooling. Start by contacting the financial aid office at any school you plan to attend to learn about scholarships, grants, and student loans. You'll find many excellent books in the public library and online resources that list various scholarships and offer tips about how to go after them. Professional associations, corporations, and other outside agencies and organizations also offer funding, much of which does not need to be paid back. Some groups will even give you additional money for living expenses. Also, many employers offer tuition reimbursement, so find out what's available where you work. There is an art and science to successfully financing your education. Funding should never be an obstacle to going back to school.

I'm too old to go back to school. If you really believe that age is an obstacle to learning, you might as well throw in the towel on life. Age is a state of mind. If you want to remain young at heart and stay fully engaged in life, get more education. You're never too old to go back to school. And if you're feeling old, school may be just the thing to rejuvenate you. Besides, everyone is living and working longer these days. Who knows what opportunities lie ahead for each of us? May as well be prepared.

I didn't enjoy my undergraduate experience, and I don't want to repeat it with graduate school. You're not alone; undergraduate school was a struggle for many of us. Part of that challenge is the volume of credits required to graduate and a diverse core curriculum of demanding subjects. Although I struggled through some classes, each course expanded my world and enriched my life in some way. However, graduate school is different. Your curriculum is more focused. Your projects and papers can be tailored to your areas of interest within your major. You have more flexibility and freedom in these studies.

Frequently Asked Questions

Besides objections, nurses often express common concerns and questions in making choices about continuing their formal education. Here are a few frequently asked questions.

Q: *Do I need to get my degrees in nursing?*

A: Earning an undergraduate or graduate nursing degree is a natural choice for some, but not for others. If teaching nursing, aspiring to advanced practice (nurse practitioner, nurse anesthetist, nurse midwife, or clinical nurse specialist), or getting a doctorate in nursing for other reasons is in your future, then a degree in nursing is the way to go. If you are working in a clinical setting such as a hospital or post-acute-care facility (subacute care, long-term acute care, etc.) or aspire to do so, a BSN or MSN degree in nursing may be required for hire or continued employment. Likewise, many school nurse positions (and some others) require a BSN for employment and for certification. Otherwise, you've got other options.

That being said, some states continue to push for a "BSN in 10" law. This would require that anyone who has an RN license in that state and graduated from an associate's degree program or hospital-based program after a certain date would be required to obtain a BSN within 10 years of graduation in order to renew their RN license past that point. Nurses who graduated prior to the law being passed might be grandfathered in and exempt from that requirement. But why take that chance? Most nurses, whether new or seasoned, would do well to simply pursue the BSN now and get it behind them. As mentioned, one option is a BSN/MSN (also called RN-to-MSN) program that allows you to work on both degrees simultaneously, potentially saving you time and money. There are even BSN-to-DNP programs for those committed to fast-tracking their education.

MY PERSONAL EDUCATIONAL JOURNEY

I was never much of a student. I scraped by during my basic education years. I just managed to struggle through a diploma in nursing program. The day I graduated, I was a happy camper, believing I would never have to sit in a classroom again.

Years later, as I contemplated what to do with the rest of my life and career, I began to think that beefing up my credentials would probably be a smart thing to do. I considered getting a degree in nursing but also explored other majors. I wasn't working in a clinical setting at the time, so I enrolled in a bachelor of science in health care management program.

I was scared to death to go back to school. Wouldn't everyone be younger and smarter than me? I wondered how long I could fool my professors into thinking I actually had something of value to contribute.

I was then amazed to learn that my fellow students were primarily my age and also working and taking care of families. We were all in the same boat. So everyone supported and helped one another.

I decided to get started and plow ahead. I couldn't think about how long it would take me, because that thought was overwhelming. I had to focus on taking one course at a time. I knew if I kept moving forward, someday I'd be finished.

When I did finally graduate several years later, I had a great sense of accomplishment. I felt more confident, more whole, and better prepared to face the world. You can't appreciate what higher education will do for you until you have it. It does change you for the better, whether you immediately recognize it or not.

Years later, I began to contemplate graduate school. I sat on the fence for years, not sure what degree I wanted to pursue. When I finally found the program I wanted to enroll in, a master's degree in corporate and public communication, I impulsively enrolled before I had much time to think about it and change my mind. I knew I was making a long-term commitment, but the way I looked at it, 5 years (the maximum amount of time the school allowed to complete the program in) would pass whether I was in school or not. At the end of those years, I could either have a graduate degree, or I could still be thinking about it. I'm glad I bit the bullet and went for it.

Remember the movie *The Wizard of Oz?* The scarecrow always felt inadequate because he didn't think he had a brain. At the end of the movie, the wizard tells him that the only difference between him and great scholars is a diploma, which he hands the scarecrow. The scarecrow, with scroll in hand, immediately begins to think great thoughts, solve complex equations, and articulate beautifully. The diploma itself didn't make the scarecrow smart. Rather, it validated something in him that allowed him to realize his full potential. That's what my graduate degree, and accompanying diploma, did for me. It validated my mental competence, and it was an empowering and emotional experience.

While in graduate school, great opportunities came my way. For example, I was asked to write a research-based article for a nursing magazine and was approached about submitting a proposal to do some consulting for a large corporation. If I had not recently learned how to do both of those things in class, I might have turned my back on those and other opportunities, feeling ill-prepared. Graduate school seemed to be preparing me for bigger and better challenges every step of the way. I always said that my formal education was the wave that was propelling me into the future. When I was finishing graduate school, people would ask me, "What are you going to do with your degree?" I'd tell them, "It's not what I'm going to do with that degree, but what that degree has already done for me."

WHERE TO FIND SCHOLARSHIP MONEY

If you're pursuing a degree in nursing or health care, contact the following sources for scholarship information:

- Your state association of the ANA (www.nursingworld.org; click on Find Your State). This applies whether you are a member or not.

- Any relevant specialty association. These could be related to your current specialty or one you intend to work in afterward. For example, if you currently work in the ICU but intend to become a certified registered nurse anesthetist, contact both the American Association of Critical-Care Nurses (AACN; www.aacn.org) and the American Association of Nurse Anesthetists (AANA; www.aana.com).

- Online nursing scholarship lists such as those referenced below. You will have to weed through them because some are designated for certain ethnic groups, levels of education, or specialties.

- Relevant ethnic heritage professional associations, if applicable, such as the National Association of Hispanic Nurses (NAHN; nahnnet. org), National Black Nurses Association Inc. (NBNA; www.nbna.org), and the Philippine Nurses Association of America Inc. (PNAA; www. mypnaa.org).

- The financial aid office in the school you are considering attending.

- *Peterson's Scholarships, Grants and Prizes (*new edition annually). This comprehensive book can be found in bookstores or the reference section of your library. Ask the librarian to help you find this and other scholarship-listing books.

- Ethnic clubs. Many have scholarship money available to those of that nationality or ethnic heritage. Similarly, some religious organizations have scholarship money available for those of the same faith.

- Philanthropic organizations, civic clubs such as Rotary Clubs, veteran's associations, unions, and organizations that support those with disabilities, if applicable.

- Your or your parent's employer, regardless of your age.

- Other business and professional associations in your community and your home state as well as the state where you will be attending college. Seek out those related to your future career plans. For example, if you are pursuing an MBA, target business and management associations.

Remember this while completing your applications:

- Applications must be filed by the deadline date and be complete. Follow the instructions carefully. Otherwise, your application will not be considered.

- Read the award criteria carefully because each scholarship has a different focus. Understand what each organization is looking for and provide relevant information.

- If you are required to write an essay, tailor your comments to the particular scholarship criteria. Choose your words carefully. Do not exceed the allowed word limit. Let the reader(s) know why this is important to you and why you are the right candidate for the award. Remember, those judging the application only have your paperwork with which to make an evaluation. Make every word count. Let your passion and commitment come through on paper. Be sure to mention any hardships, challenges, or special circumstances, such as being a single parent, disabled person, veteran, first generation American, immigrant, sole supporter of your family, or recipient of special recognition or honors received in the past.

- Just like a résumé, your application should be free of spelling, grammar, and punctuation errors. A typed application makes a good impression.

- The more scholarships you apply for, the better your chances of receiving awards. Some organizations even award money for living expenses in addition to tuition.

Where to find scholarship listings:

- Discover Nursing: www.discovernursing.com and MinorityNurse.com.

- Sigma (formerly Sigma Theta Tau International): www.sigmanursing. org/advance-elevate/careers/nursing-scholarship-opportunities.

- The Foundation of the National Association of Student Nurses (FNSNA): www.forevernursing.org.

- Generic listings can be found on sites such as fastweb.com.

- Start filling out the applications, writing the essays, and sticking on the stamps or hitting the enter button. Money, or lack of it, should never be an excuse not to go back to school. Where there is a will there is always a way! There is definitely money out there for you. Go after it.

Q: *Because I came into nursing with a degree in another major, why do I still need to get a BSN or MSN? Isn't my nonnursing degree(s) recognized?*

A: Many individuals are coming to the profession from a prior career or after a nonnursing college course of study. If you enter via an associate nursing degree program, a BSN or MSN will be a natural next step for most. While your nonnursing degrees do have value and will be recognized as part of your professional package, they are not a substitute for a degree in nursing in the situations mentioned above under "Do I need to get my degrees in nursing?" There is evidence of improved patient outcomes in studying nursing theory, research, and concepts and their applications, as well as health promotion, policy, ethics, and economics, all of which are part of a nursing major curriculum.

Baby-boomer nurse Katarina graduated from nursing school in 1975. She has worked in the same hospital and in the same department since then. She lamented to me, "I'm stuck here because I don't have my bachelor's degree. I know I'll have trouble finding a job anywhere else without it. I don't plan to retire any time soon but don't want to keep doing the same thing indefinitely." I told her that she could easily get unstuck by enrolling in school and getting started on the process, one course at a time. I even gave her scholarship resources. I'm happy to report that with a little prodding and support she is now pursuing her BSN in her 60s. She tells me that while it is challenging balancing family, work, and school, she feels reenergized in her career and looks forward to the future.

Q: *Which degree will give me the best job prospects and the highest earning potential?*

A: No one degree is right for every situation. If you interview hospital, health care, and nursing administrators and managers, you'll discover that they have degrees in different majors. If you talk to other successful nurses, you'll discover that some have degrees in nursing and others in diverse majors such as health care administration, business, education, communication, public health, and even journalism. Some schools offer a dual MSN-MBA. That's a great combo since today's nurse needs to be as much a business person as a clinician.

No college degree alone will ever guarantee career success. That is largely up to you. Which degree you pursue is an individual choice based on your career goals and interests. Your best bet is to choose a course of study that interests and excites you and then find a way to make it work for you. We'll talk more about the decision-making process and clarifying career goals in chapter 3.

Q: *There are so many choices for nursing graduate degrees, how do I know which one to choose?*

A: There are more education options than ever today. This can be both exciting and overwhelming, not to mention confusing, at the same time. It's important to first decide whether or not advanced practice is something you want to pursue. That decision should not be taken lightly as it requires a commitment to taking your practice to the next level and then maintaining that level once you get there. Be sure to do an informational interview (see chapter 3) with several others successfully practicing in that advanced role and specialty before deciding. There's also the clinical nurse leader (CNL) track for those nurses who wish to take their practice to the next level without becoming an advanced practice nurse (APN).

However, there are many other options including an MSN in education, administration, informatics, and so on. Which major you choose when pursuing an MSN is less important than actually obtaining the MSN. As mentioned above, choose the program with course work and curriculum that is most appealing to you. If you obtain an MSN in administration, that will not preclude you from going after positions in nursing education. Nor will an MSN in nursing informatics be a barrier to your pursing nursing administration roles and so on. The MSN after your name is what really matters.

Q: *Are online programs as good as traditional programs?*

A: If an online program is appropriately accredited, it shares the same legitimacy as a traditional one. Since online degrees are so prevalent today, even at the doctoral level, they are widely accepted. Both distance learning and traditional classroom learning have their advantages and disadvantages. Fully explore both options before choosing the one that's right for you. It is helpful to talk to students who have completed both online and traditional classroom-based programs before deciding what's right for you. Every student has different needs and interests.

Q: *Where can I find more information about schools, majors, and accreditation status?*

A: A few sources of information include the National League for Nursing (NLN; www.nln.org), AACN (www.aacn.nche.edu), the *College Blue Book* found in the reference section of a library, and Peterson's *Graduate and Professional Programs* and other Peterson's guides (www.petersons.com).

> For those with a bachelor's degree in another major wishing to enter the nursing profession, accelerated and second-degree BSN programs exist. These are typically 12–18 months in length. Some prerequisite courses may be required before entering. And because of the rigorous class and clinical schedule, some schools may discourage or even prohibit working while attending.

Ongoing Education and Training

In addition to formal education, there are many other opportunities to keep your brain sharp. Here are just a few.

Participate in continuing education. You may live in a state that requires CE in the form of a certain number of contact hours for license renewal. Aside from that, CE should be a way of life for a professional. Opportunities abound for sanctioned nursing CE through seminars and classes, print publications, and online sources.

But there are plenty of other avenues for ongoing learning, too. See what's offered through your local adult school programs. Many colleges and universities offer noncredit courses and certificate programs in various subjects. Don't restrict your learning to clinical topics. Work on improving your skills in communication, writing, public speaking, and anything else that interests you or can enhance your knowledge, skill set, or expertise.

Work on your computer skills. Computers are an integral part of our life and work. If you don't already feel comfortable using computers and navigating your way around the Internet, take steps to get up to speed or you'll be left behind. Although computers are still intimidating to some, once you master the basics, your confidence level will soar. You'll also be more marketable.

Make a commitment to stay up to date with new programs, platforms, and software. Adult schools and community colleges have classes for computer users from beginner to advanced levels. Many public libraries offer free related courses. If you prefer to learn in the privacy of your own home, hire a computer tutor. Experienced friends and family members can be a great help and are usually happy to assist.

Get social media savvy. Social media (Facebook, LinkedIn, Twitter, etc.) is a dominant means of communication in our society and not just for social purposes. Nor is it just for the "young," as some folks believe. Social media (SM) is used in most workplaces and professional circles for communicating, networking, ongoing education, marketing, job finding and recruiting, and more. Many workplaces and educational institutions use SM for online communication rather than email. But it is also an important place to have a professional presence.

If you're not yet SM savvy, start working to get up to speed. Engage in self-learning, get a friend or colleague to help you, or hire a SM consultant to get you set up and advise you how to use it for professional purposes.

Get to the library. That's right, the good old brick-and-mortar public library. Your local library is a vast source of almost totally free information. You can find books and multimedia products that address any subject under the sun. Whether you want to learn about Medicare regulations, how to write an article for publication, or acquire management skills, you'll find plentiful resources. Be sure to check out the audio books and educational videos, too. Plus, libraries typically have access to all the major online research and other databases that you can access for free even from home once you have a library card.

College and health care center libraries are great resources. With very few exceptions, both allow the general public to use their facilities. Of course, you might not be able to take any books out if you're not a student, employee, or alumnus there, but you can read, photocopy, research, and take notes as needed. If you use the library of a university that offers degrees in nursing, you'll likely find a vast number of nursing and health care journals in their periodicals section. If your employer has a library, talk to the health sciences librarian to help you with whatever you need or want to learn. Most nurses underutilize this resource.

Don't hesitate to ask the librarian or research assistant to help you find what you're looking for, either online or in the stacks. That's what they're there for and are generally willing to help you. Utilize this source when working on school-related projects, developing a work-related in-service, writing an article for publication, or preparing to speak or present a poster at a conference.

Get certified in your specialty. If you have a few years of experience in a particular specialty and think you might continue to work in that area, look into getting certified. Certification based on experience and education is a measure of competency and a standard of excellence. It gives you higher standards to strive for in your practice and will, in many cases, make you more marketable. It also instills pride and a sense of confidence. Many health care facilities now post on individual units the names and photos of nurses who are certified in that specialty. This instills confidence in patients and their loved ones as well as demonstrating that nurses can specialize and be board certified just as physicians are. Clinical certification is usually one component of a clinical ladder program as well.

Get a grip on the big picture. Nurses have a tendency to focus solely on their current specialty. That's fine to a point, but you have got to broaden your knowledge base of the bigger issues that affect nursing and health care as well as the world around you. How can you effectively plan your career and know what specialties will be in demand if you are not aware of the trends and issues that will shape future health care and nursing?

Find out what health care economists are predicting for the next 5–10 years. Learn about the concept of universal health care and its possible effects on the workplace. Everyone in health care is talking about mandated nurse-to-patient staffing ratios. Are you fully aware of the pros and cons? Get the facts so you have an informed opinion.

Where can you find all this information? It's just a few computer clicks away. Use the Internet to search for related topics, using key phrases such as "health care industry forecasts" and "nursing career trends." Spend some time in the library (including your employer's library if applicable) and online reading health care and nursing news magazines, such as *Nurse.com, Nursing Economic$, Modern Healthcare, Hospitals & Health Networks*, and *Journal of Nursing Administration*. Challenge your brain and expand your perspective with mainstream newspapers and news magazines as well, whether print or online.

Casting a Wide Net

Networking is one of the most important activities you can do for personal and professional success. It's all about connections. It's about meeting new people and developing relationships as well as staying in touch with those you already know. Think of your network as a support team, an information pipeline, a safety net, and a personal think tank all in one. Networking allows you to tap into the collective wisdom, experience, and connections of those in your community, which in this communication age is often virtual and can include almost anyone in the universe.

While some people think of networking as someone of importance pulling strings for you, it is actually a reciprocal process of giving and getting information and support. Networking is an interactive two-way street. Under the best circumstances, it is mutually beneficial.

Networking is misunderstood and highly underused by nurses. Why are we so reluctant to develop a network? Maybe because of the confidential nature of the work we do. We've become so accustomed to staying quiet that we're often reluctant to talk to others. Some of us are rusty with our socialization skills. Others may feel competitive and insecure, believing it's better to tough it out on their own, rather than giving and receiving help and support. Some nurses think that everyday networking is superficial and pointless. I recently heard a nurse say, "I can't see the purpose of schmoozing just for schmoozing's sake." However, networking helps everyone involved, and it enables them to help even more people. It always has a purpose, even if only to stay connected to people you already know or to meet new people. One of the very exciting things about networking is that you never know whom you're going to meet or run into.

By effectively developing and using a network, you can:

- Achieve your goals more quickly;
- Stay completely up-to-date on issues and information;
- Be more effective in your current job;
- Share ideas and information;
- Increase your chances of getting a promotion or breaking into a particular specialty;
- Get additional and secondary contacts to expand your network;
- Find out about a company, a specific job, or a specialty;
- Get introductions to industry leaders, decision-makers, and other influential people;
- Discover hidden jobs that exist in a company that are not publicly advertised; and
- Develop a "virtual" support system that goes where you go.

Where can you network? Out of all the different ways to network, face-to-face networking is the most effective. When you meet someone in person, you get a face to go with the name and have the opportunity to share a handshake and make eye contact. You get a sense of who the person is and vice versa. In-person encounters are generally more productive and memorable. Likewise, periodically seeing the people you know is always better than merely keeping in touch through other distant or online means. There is greater opportunity for interaction and communication. Below are some good places for face-to-face networking.

Professional association meetings. I've already mentioned the benefits of being active in professional associations, but your network should expand beyond nursing and even beyond health care. Consider attending an occasional chamber of commerce meeting, associations of professional business people, and other health care professions' meetings. You don't need to be a member of an organization or even work in a particular field to attend a few meetings as a guest.

Ask a few colleagues what organizations they belong to and ask to tag along to a meeting. It's always easier to go with someone you know, especially the first time. However, you have to make a point to talk to at least one new person while you're there, or you defeat the purpose of going from a networking perspective.

Career fairs. Contrary to popular belief, career fairs are not just for job seekers. They're a great place to meet people and stay in touch with those you already know. In addition to the array of employers exhibiting, schools of higher learning are usually represented as well, along with an occasional publisher, medical product company, and other vendors. A potential added benefit is a wide array of CE programs offered on such diverse subjects as stress management, bioterrorism, public speaking skills, and clinical topics.

Some career fairs are for nursing, some are for the health care industry in general, and others are for a specific industry, such as the pharmaceutical industry. Other job fairs are general in nature and include companies in the health care business or outside it. You never know whom you'll meet at these events, what companies will be represented, and what opportunities will be available. Even if you're content working where you are, you should always be exploring your options. Besides, *the best time to look for your next job is while you're happily employed.*

If you're worried someone will see you there and tell your boss, who may in turn think that you're looking for another job, solve that problem by telling your boss beforehand that you're going. You might say you're contemplating going back to school and want to talk to the educational exhibitors who will be there. You can also say you want to attend the CE programs sometimes offered at job fairs.

Conventions. You don't have to be a member of an organization to attend its convention. Many conventions offer special registration options for one day versus the entire event. I once attended a medical convention with a friend who is a physician. I had a blast. I attended a workshop on health care reimbursement issues and discovered I knew more about the subject than most of the physicians in the audience. I also attended a workshop there on dressing well for my body type and coloring. I found it very helpful.

ASKING FOR HELP

Years ago, when I was hired as director of DRG services, I was told that I'd eventually be responsible for the quality improvement (QI) department. I had no experience in that specialty whatsoever.

When the time came for me to organize that department, I got on the telephone and called several area hospitals and asked to speak with their director of QI. I introduced myself and asked for their help. I asked what I should do first, what associations I should join, what key issues I needed to know about, and if they could share a copy of their policy and procedure manual. Everyone was gracious and eager to help. We all stayed in touch after that and exchanged information and resources. We created a local network that was mutually supportive and beneficial.

Alumni events. Alumni have an immediate camaraderie with one another and a special bond, regardless of their year of graduation or their major. And since many alumni have great connections and influence, it pays to stay in touch. Use your alumnus status as a connection. Don't hesitate to mention it in conversation or in correspondence as appropriate. It immediately builds trust. You might, for example, find out via LinkedIn or other means that a director of nursing or chief executive officer (CEO) of a particular health care system is a fellow graduate of your school. Utilize that connection.

Seminars and educational programs. When you attend educational activities outside of your workplace, you can network with the speakers, the attendees, and those running the event. But don't ignore others in the vicinity. Whenever I attend any type of meeting or event at a hotel or conference center, I always scan the schedule to see who else is meeting there. I have often stopped in on another meeting to meet the event organizers or speakers during their breaks. The opportunities are endless when you get yourself out there.

Community activities. Get out to the occasional political rally, school board meeting, church social, or school fair. Even block parties provide great networking opportunities. You'll be amazed at the information you'll gather and the connections you'll make as well as what you learn about others as you let them into your circle—even casual acquaintances. Find a way to mention in conversation if you're job hunting, starting a business, or interested in breaking into a particular specialty or working for a particular company or agency. That type of self-revelation can help to uncover hidden resources in your own backyard.

Anywhere there are people. Once you develop a networking mindset and become accustomed to talking to people, you'll be amazed at the interesting people you'll meet and run into virtually anywhere. I have met celebrities, CEOs, famous authors, and many interesting nurses and others on trains, planes, shuttle buses, and in the beauty parlor!

Increasing Your Networking Opportunities

To stay current with meetings and other related activities, view event calendars in nursing magazines and web sites. Check out the community events calendar in your local newspaper. Ask colleagues to keep you informed of upcoming meetings and conferences and to pass on brochures to you. You can also contact various organizations and ask to be put on their traditional and email mailing lists. Sites like Meetup and Eventbrite can also help locate events of interest to you.

The Internet is a great networking tool. Connect on social media such as LinkedIn and Twitter, join Facebook and LinkedIn groups and other online nursing communities, and join in on the occasional live chat. These are all forums for sharing information and ideas, garnering support, making initial contacts, staying in touch, and keeping up with what's happening. You can sometimes find these forums and groups listed on professional association, general nursing, and career web sites or by doing an Internet search for "nursing discussion forums" or "Facebook nurse groups" and so on.

While email is not an appropriate form of communication in every situation, it is a fast, easy way to stay in touch with some people and to make preliminary contact with someone before calling them. It can also serve as an introduction or provide easy access to influential people. You can even reach the White House via email. Don't rely exclusively on SM messaging for initial (or any) contacts since many people do not check those messages. Email is still more reliable in many cases.

That being said, there's still nothing like picking up the telephone and actually talking to someone. In fact, if you are accustomed to emailing someone all the time, be sure to occasionally speak with them by phone. It's more personal and interactive. And some people find it easier to speak by phone than to type a response through email.

Of course there's always the US Postal Service (USPS). Traditional mail or "snail mail" is a great way to stay in touch, too, through the use of greeting cards or an occasional handwritten note to say "Thanks" or "Congratulations." In this electronic age, people appreciate the personal, low-tech forms of communication.

Usual Objections to Networking
Just as a litany of excuses is used as justification for not joining organizations or continuing education, networking detractors have raised their own unworthy objections.

I don't have time to network. We all have schedules that seem maxed out. We all feel tired and overwhelmed. The amazing thing is that face-to-face networking can energize you. The connections you make, the interesting people you meet, the support and energy you gather, and the ideas and information you pick up through networking stimulate you. Networking also lessens your feelings of being alone, helping you feel upbeat and hopeful with a sense of being part of a greater whole.

I can't get out of the house. Maybe your work schedule or childcare issues prevent you from attending formal networking events. Try to make arrangements beforehand to get the time off or have someone help you out at home. Even if you can't get out, formal events are not the only place to network. We all come in contact with people at work, at the grocery store, through our children's school, and through social activities. Opportunities exist everywhere. Remember, networking is not confined to nursing and health care circles. Additionally, you always have the Internet, telephone, and USPS.

LinkedIn

LinkedIn (LI) is the most important social network for professionals. It provides an opportunity to create an online portfolio showcasing current and previous employment, education, credentials, endorsements, recommendations, and more. LI is used by prospective employers and recruiters to find and screen job candidates. It is also used by prospective clients to find consultants and vendors. But whether you are actively seeking employment or clients or not, LI is a place to make valuable connections to expand and maintain your network, make and get introductions to other professionals, exchange ideas and information, and build credibility and visibility. As already stated, a professional online presence is vital in today's digital world.

Many (if not most) employers automatically search for a LI profile when receiving a résumé or after meeting at a career event. In fact some employers are more interested in a candidate's LI profile (because it can be more comprehensive in some ways) than a résumé. If you don't have a LI profile, or if you do and it is incomplete or not up-to-date, you put yourself at a great disadvantage and may be discounted. It is also common for professionals, after meeting you, to automatically go to LI to connect and learn more about you. It's become so significant in professional circles that many people post their LinkedIn URL on their business cards and résumés along with their email address.

If you don't have a LI account yet, open one. A basic account—all you need to get started—is free. If necessary, find someone familiar with the network and ask them to help you set yours up and use it to your best advantage. You can also hire a social media consultant to help. Once you have an account, start working on your profile and keep it up to date. Next, join some groups there that are of interest to you. Contribute occasionally by sharing an opinion or pertinent information and responding to group discussions and questions. All of this will serve to demonstrate your expertise, become better known, and garner the attention of important and influential people.

Search for others to connect with including current and past supervisors and coworkers, those you meet through various networking channels, and individuals that you'd like to get to know better. It's ideal to send a personal note with your online invitation to connect on LI to let others (who might not know you or recognize your name) know why you are inviting them to connect. You might simply say, "I enjoy your posts and would like to stay connected on LI." Or "I see that we both attended XYZ University. I graduated in 2006 from the nursing program. I'd love to be connected here."

I'm too shy and nervous. If you don't get out much, as many nurses do not, your socialization skills get rusty. Of course, some of us may not have been very good at networking to begin with. There are certainly those who seem to be able to work a room like a pro, but they have usually learned and practiced their networking skills out of necessity or desire. The truth is, most people consider themselves shy networkers.

Many people are uncomfortable socializing because they have trouble remembering people's names. They may be uncomfortable making conversation, or they may not know how to break the ice with strangers. These are skills that can be learned and mastered with a little know-how and practice.

Networking is a pervasive theme throughout this book because it's very important. This section serves merely as an introduction to the whys and wheres of networking. The how-tos and other important uses for networking will be discussed in more depth in subsequent chapters.

Chapter 3

Where Do I Go from Here?

While some nurses have a clear idea of where they want to be 5 years from now, many do not. I frequently hear nurses say, "I don't know what I want to be when I grow up," and these are not necessarily young nurses. Most of us just keep doing what we've been doing without much thought about or planning for our future. It's so easy to get stuck in a rut. That's when what you do ceases to become a career and becomes just a job.

Many people are under the mistaken belief that if they don't know what they want to do, they can't move forward until they make that decision. On the contrary, you have to start moving forward, creating some momentum in your professional life, discover what you're good at, where your special talents and interests lie, and where the opportunities are. Indecision won't solve anything. It will only magnify self-doubt and anxiety.

While some nurses do exactly the same thing for years on end, others haphazardly hop around from job to job on an eternal quest to find their niche. They often do this, unfortunately, without considering what they enjoy doing, what they're good at, or what their ideal work environment might be. When they don't take time to explore their own wants and needs and get in tune with their strengths and assets, they waste a lot of time looking for career satisfaction in a place of employment, rather than looking for that satisfaction within themselves. Instead, they should think about their own interests and then look for a position that supports those interests, rather than taking any job that comes along hoping they'll discover it will suit them.

All About You

As nurses, we are versatile and multitalented, but we are notorious for underestimating our own value and capabilities. We are good at many different things. These abilities are so second nature to us that we may not see them as assets. We are so accustomed to doing whatever comes our way that we lose sight of how creative, skillful, and knowledgeable we are at handling it.

So what exactly are we good at?

We are master multitaskers. We juggle so many balls at one time, and we're not juggling lightweight Styrofoam balls either; it's more like keeping a chain saw, a flaming torch, a live chicken, and a fragile piece of china in the air. I used to tell prospective employers that for every year I worked in the hospital, I got 2 years' worth of experience. I was making a point about how the work, responsibilities, and new knowledge I acquired on an ongoing basis, as well as the actions I had to initiate in the drama of a typical nurse's day, were worth more than their weight in time.

Nurses are organized, detail oriented, and acutely aware of their surroundings. We think on our feet, making quick decisions and managing complex projects. We're excellent problem solvers and are totally customer service oriented. Nurses possess excellent communication skills. We regularly translate complex medical material into terms that can be understood by the variety of people with whom we interact. We often adjust our language and our style of speaking from moment to moment without conscious thought, communicating with an array of people, from those with big egos to those under extreme stress. And we have to do this with a culturally diverse population.

Here is a partial list of strengths and assets of the average nurse:

Skills

Analyzing	Decision-making
Communicating effectively	Developing programs
Counseling and coaching	Managing time

Organizing

Planning

Presenting and speaking

Problem solving

Researching

Selling (yes, selling! I elaborate below)

Supervising and managing

Teaching and training

Team leading

Writing reports

Attributes

Adaptable

Creative

Dependable

Detail oriented

Flexible

Hardworking

Innovative

Independent

People oriented

Reliable

Resourceful

Responsible

Sense of humor

Team player

Thinks on their feet

Works well under pressure

In addition to the talents and abilities that nurses use every day in traditional health care settings, they also possess many skills that can be transferred to other areas of practice. For example, nurses are natural teachers. We instruct all the time without thinking about it. And we are engaged in public speaking, which is nothing more than teaching on a grander scale.

Nurses are natural salespeople, too. We have to "sell" constantly in the clinical setting. Every time you have to convince a patient to adhere to a regimen or follow up on a test, you are selling. An even harder sell is when you have to convince a member of the health care team that something is a good idea when they don't see it that way. You are pointing out the benefits to the buyer, overcoming objections, and closing the sale. We do that every day in nursing. These skills are easily transferable to sales of health products, pharmaceuticals, and services.

Nurses also possess a great body of knowledge and experience that is very valuable and transferable to many settings including legal nurse consulting, research, writing, and consulting. Remember when I was offered the position of center manager at the weight control center and was convinced I couldn't do it? I quickly learned that my nursing instincts, assessment skills, decision-making capabilities, brains, and prior experience had actually prepared me well for the business world. But of course, at the time, I still had that "just a nurse" mentality.

Self-Assessment

A fundamental first step in developing a career plan is to do an honest self-assessment. This is not something you can develop in an hour. You need some time to think about it, reflect on past experiences, and talk with those who know you well. Get a notebook, legal pad, or a journal, or sit at your computer. Write down or type the following questions. Then take some time to ponder the answers and write down your thoughts. It may take you a month or more to compile an accurate profile. It is important to write these things down and not just think about them. Why? Because putting pen to paper or fingers to keyboard takes something from the abstract and makes it concrete. It helps to clarify your thoughts and desires. It gives you a visual reference to read, reread, and rewrite.

Question 1: What Do I Enjoy Doing?

Does the challenge of hands-on care make your heart beat faster? Do you love teaching and working with students and new hires? Is writing something you have a passion for? Are you interested more in the big picture of things—project management, budget development, and staffing studies? Does public policy excite you? Write down anything that makes you feel excited or challenged, that feeds your creative side, or that gives you satisfaction. It doesn't matter whether you think you can make a living at it, think it is practical for you, or think you're "any good" at it. Just write it down. Many of us never take the time to think about what we really enjoy doing, yet that should be at the heart of everything we do in our career.

If you're still not sure what you enjoy, become more self-aware in your everyday work. What parts of your job do you enjoy the most and the least? Think about things you've done in the past that have given you satisfaction and enjoyment. And by the way, it doesn't have to be strictly related to nursing and health care. Many a nurse has combined their nursing career with a seemingly unrelated interest such as flying, sports, music, the outdoors, and even farming.

Question 2: What Am I Good At?

Each of us has special talents and abilities. Certain things come easy to us or seem to be natural. Others admire us for certain traits and often seek our advice or help on related issues. Is there something people have complimented you on or told you you're good at, whether you agree with them or not?

If you're not sure what you do well, or even if you think you *do* know what you do well, ask a few people who know you what they see as your strong points. You may be pleasantly surprised by the responses you get and discover something or some things positive about yourself. Often our strong points are so much a part of who we are that we do not necessarily see them. In other words, we take them for granted.

Question 3: What Am I Interested In?

Maybe you've been curious to learn more about computers and how they work in health care. Perhaps you're intrigued by a different specialty or type of employer. Or have you ever thought you'd like to learn more about holistic healing and wellness? Maybe the law has always fascinated you, and you've wondered if that field might be right for you. Write down everything you can think of, putting those that intrigue you most at the top.

Many nurses have told me they have absolutely no idea what they want to do or what they're interested in. Yet, when pressed, there is often something hovering just below the surface. I once spoke with a nurse who was frantically trying to change her career, but she couldn't identify any special interests. I took the conversation in another direction and she revealed that she loved to write and had always wanted to pursue that. When I pointed out that she had just revealed something she actually did have a strong interest in, she snapped, "Nobody makes any money at that." In reality, there are many nurses making a part- or full-time living by writing.

However, many of us resist our own thoughts and desires because of fears, preconceived notions about ourselves and other things, and expectations that we, our family, and our friends have of us. Everyone dreams about something, whether they want to admit it or not. Sometimes the dream is so well hidden and buried so deep that we even forget it exists.

Question 4: What Transferable Skills Do I Have?

Ask yourself, "What have I done? What are my experiences?" Transferable skills are those practices you have experience with that can be used in alternate settings or in alternative ways. Nurses have a tendency to focus solely on their clinical skills. However, as previously mentioned, nurses are excellent at many other things. Focus on any business or managerial experience you've had, such as working on schedules or budgets. Do you ever take a charge position or supervisory role on your unit, even if only occasionally? How about working with students or new hires? Have you developed an educational tool or fact sheet? Have you presented at grand rounds, presented in-services, or been a liaison to outside agencies? Do you love technology?

Question 5: What Areas Do I Need and Want to Improve In?

Maybe you need to get an updated look in terms of your hairstyle and clothing; we all get in ruts with our appearance as well as our work. Perhaps your communication skills need some work. Maybe you need to expand your computer skills, become more adept at using social media, or advance your formal education. You might need to find some creative outlets or down time to create some balance and harmony in your life. Write down whatever you can think of. Focus on both professional and personal things since the two go hand in hand.

Years ago, I received a call from a distraught nurse. She had just gone on an interview for a position she really wanted and was turned down for the job. She felt lost and deflated and was looking for guidance. She told me she had been an oncology nurse for 15 years and had applied for a position to do some counseling for a new program being started by a pharmaceutical company. The prospective employer had seen her résumé and called her in for an interview. I asked her how the interview went, and she said she thought it went well.

This nurse proceeded to tell me that she made it clear to the interviewer that she didn't have any counseling experience. She further advised them that she was willing to learn and take any courses they wanted to send her to, but again emphasized she didn't have any experience. In reality, this nurse had 15 years of counseling experience as an oncology nurse. She just didn't see it. Instead, she went to great lengths to talk her way out of a job. This is one very unfortunate example of how nurses are often unable to identify innate skills and abilities and transfer them to other areas of practice.

Question 6: What Would My Ideal Work Environment Be Like?

Think about the type of environment you'd like to work in and the parameters of your work life. For example, would you prefer a patient care area, a traditional business setting, or a home-based office? Would you prefer to be stationary, or would you like to be on the road sometimes? Would you prefer to work regular business hours or have flexible scheduling that might include weekends and holidays, or do shift work? Are you looking for 12-hour shifts, part-time work, or a per diem position?

Finding Your Niche

Now that you've done your self-assessment, you still don't know what you want to be when you grow up, right? Again, that's normal for most of us. Many nurses get so hung up on finding what they believe is that one right job or specialty, the elusive niche, that they forget to savor the process of getting there. You've probably heard the expression, "Success is a journey, not a destination." That means you have to focus more on the process and less on the outcome.

Catherine says, "I often push myself to try new things in order to step out of my personal boundaries and to learn more about myself. It seems that most people don't understand their own strengths and weaknesses until they compare themselves to others or until they put themselves in a completely new and different situation. When I attend professional association meetings, get involved in a new project, or try my hand at something new, I realize my own good qualities and shortcomings more clearly."

I'm always amazed when I hear a new graduate nervously say they haven't found their niche yet, when they've barely started their career. We put such pressure on ourselves to discover our place. Some of us think we'll have a revelation of sorts. In reality, that "niche" will likely change from time to time and will evolve as you move forward, especially since we're all living and working longer than in the past. As you read in chapter 1, I tried on many hats before getting where I am today. Have I reached my final career destination yet? I doubt it. I'm still a traveler.

In order to focus on the process, you need actions and activities that will lead you down a path of discovery about yourself, your opportunities, and the world around you. Keep in mind that you don't need to know exactly where you're headed or exactly what you want to do in order to get on with your life and career. However, by moving in a positive, forward direction, the right path will eventually reveal itself to you. In other words, you've got to move forward in faith. Ideas, inspiration, and enlightenment come from the most unexpected sources and in the most unexpected ways and places. That's why it's important to create momentum in your professional life. Here are ways to do just that.

Accumulate Experiences

There are lots of opportunities to stretch yourself in your professional life. By trying new things, you may find something you like or something you're good at. You'll also learn more about the bigger world of nursing and health care in general. These are all necessary steps to developing a career path.

Offer to work on special projects at work. Try your hand at doing the schedule or department budget. Take a shot at being a preceptor to students and new nurses. Make yourself available to attend recruitment events or work at community health-screening programs. Propose a department QI project and offer to conduct the research and write up the report. Get appointed to a shared governance council. These, and other related activities, will expose you to new things and force you to develop new skills. By the way, I'm not suggesting you do these things out of a sense of loyalty to your employer, rather, I'm suggesting you do these things because of what's in it for you.

Get on facility-wide committees. Find some interprofessional (or interdepartmental) committees that interest you (such as a recruitment and retention, QI, or safety committee) and volunteer to be a part of them. Getting on these committees is a good way to pick up new skills and experiences, expand your knowledge base, increase your influence, develop new relationships, and learn something about yourself in the process. Plus, many departmental and system-wide problems are solved at the committee level. This gives you an opportunity to have your voice heard and be part of the solution rather than part of the problem.

Use Professional Associations as Training Grounds

Hopefully, I made a good case for why you should join and become active in professional associations in chapter 2. But again, you never know how or where those experiences will work out for you.

When I launched my education business years ago, I started out by offering public seminars in my home state and later across the country. People would often ask me, "How did you ever learn to run seminars like that? How did you know what to do?" I responded, "Believe it or not, I learned while I was the education chair for a state professional association I belonged to years ago. We ran an annual full-day seminar. I had to negotiate with national speakers, contract with hotels, apply for continuing education credits, work with a graphic designer and printer to develop a brochure, market the program, and coordinate all on-site activities the day of the event." Did I envision myself someday running my own seminars back then? The thought never occurred to me. But Benjamin Disraeli once said, "The secret of success in life is for a man to be ready for his opportunity when it comes." So how can you prepare for something that hasn't happened yet? When an opportunity presents itself, consider it and think about what you might be able to learn to prepare for future opportunities rather than being so quick to say no.

Bob was an ICU nurse who was interested in learning new things. When his manager asked for a volunteer to sit on a new hospital-wide communication committee, Bob jumped at the chance: "I thought it sounded interesting so I agreed to participate." He asked how much time would be required and was told 2–3 hours per month, which he could do on work time. The purpose of the committee was to evaluate how the various departments received and transmitted information. The committee would then be asked to make suggestions for improvement.

One of the recommendations that came from the committee was for the hospital to install a computerized patient-charting system. Part of the proposal included creating a new full-time position to oversee the project installation, train all current and future employees, act as liaison to the hardware and software vendors, and be a troubleshooter. Once the proposal was approved, whom do you think they offered that job to? Bob became the hospital's first nursing informatics specialist and has never looked back. Bob's experience can be summed up with a line from *A Hero in Every Heart* by H. Jackson Brown Jr. (1996, 43): "Opportunity dances with those who are already on the dance floor."

Showcase Your Special Talents and Interests

If you like to write, volunteer to work on the employee newsletter or develop some patient education materials. If you love to teach and speak, volunteer to present at grand rounds, do department in-services, or provide some community education. If technology is your cup of tea, offer to create a database for scheduling or QI data. Show the world what you're capable of doing and develop your special talents at the same time.

Patti Rager, RN, is former president and publisher of Nursing Spectrum (now known as Nurse.com), a communications and publishing company.

Early in her nursing career, Patti took the initiative to develop her love of writing:

> *I started newsletters for the nursing department and the community as a sideline in two consecutive hospital positions I held. After I completed my MBA, I took courses in a magazine certificate program. I was then recruited to launch the Nursing Spectrum magazine in Washington, DC. Little did I know that I had been 'practicing' to later become president and publisher of Nursing Spectrum! You never know what nurses will end up doing.*

Use Volunteering as a Career Management Tool

Many people think of volunteering as something charitable you do to help others. Although that may be true, there are also many benefits to the volunteer. If you'd like to get some teaching experience, doing that as a volunteer for a social service organization like the American Red Cross or American Heart Association is a smart thing to do. Would you like experience organizing public events or using information technology? Volunteering your services to a clinic or local public health agency is a great way to get it. Volunteer experience is no less valid or meaningful than paid experience. It's wonderful to volunteer for altruistic reasons, but always look for the opportunities and consider the potential for personal growth in any situation.

Explore Career Options

The majority of nurses are not aware of the broad scope of opportunities that are available to them both in and out of the hospital. Not only do most nurses lack knowledge about various options, but they often have inaccurate preconceived notions about certain specialties and positions based on outdated or incorrect information.

Even if you're happy in your current specialty, it's important to know what options are out there. Knowing you have options lessens your anxiety about the future. Each nurse should understand the full scope of what other nurses are doing. Here are some ways to explore career options.

Attend related seminars and workshops. Programs on specific specialties as well as general career option programs are offered by colleges, professional associations, communication companies, and private education companies.

Get out to career fairs. These events generally offer presentations on specific career opportunities. Not only can you learn something, you can also talk with the speaker and others actually doing that thing. You can also discuss various types of career offerings with exhibitors.

Spend time online. You'll find general nursing sites and related professional association web sites with tons of information and resources about various specialties. You'll also find articles, webinars, live chats, and more. Use search phrases such as "nursing career specialties," "nursing specialties," "career alternatives for nurses," "nontraditional nursing specialties," and "trends in nursing careers [current year]."

Talk to other nurses. Talk to the nurses you meet at meetings, in your workplace, or in other situations. Ask them to tell you about what they do.

Attend some specialty professional association meetings as a guest. If you're considering working in the operating room (OR), for example, attend a local chapter meeting of the Association of periOperative Registered Nurses (AORN) as a guest. Tag along with a friend or go by yourself.

Counselors and Coaches

Sometimes a qualified professional can help you in your journey. Such a person can serve as an objective third party to help you identify your strengths, explore options, decide where you fit in, help you effectively market yourself, and work on specific problems and challenges. They will not place you in a job as an employment agency or professional recruiter might, but they will assist you in that process.

Career counselors have a graduate degree in counseling and specialized education and training in career management. They must be licensed or certified. Many career counselors use standardized testing to identify personality traits and interests. These tests don't actually tell you what type of career or specialty you should be in, but rather they tell you what fields people with similar traits are working in. Some career counselors can also help you develop a career plan and clarify career goals. They can be particularly helpful if you have specific personal or career challenges to deal with, such as a spotty work history, a disability, or a history of addiction.

Career coaches don't need to be licensed, although some are certified by professional associations. They do some of the same things that a career counselor does, depending on their background and expertise. A coach might be characterized as a catalyst, a facilitator, or a personal trainer for career-related issues. Like a career counselor, they can help you decide what's right for you and then help you get there. They can give you specific advice that will help you clarify goals, develop an action plan, and then hold you accountable to meet those goals.

Joan, a registered nurse and life and career coach, offers this definition of coaching: "The goal of coaching is to support and partner with you to move toward the goals that are meaningful to you, and away from what is holding you back. By focusing on the action steps you can take in the present, a coach helps you create the future you want."

If you seek the services of a coach or counselor for help with your career, consider one who is also a nurse. A nurse career coach or counselor has unique insights into the special skills and abilities and psyches of nurses and should be familiar with the vast array of opportunities out there for nurses. Those outside of nursing sometimes hold a limited view of what we do and lack in-depth knowledge about related opportunities and assume that an unhappy bedside nurse needs to find a new profession.

Where can you find these people? The best way to find a competent career professional is through word of mouth or personal referrals. In other words, ask around. You may be able to get a referral through a nursing or health care professional association including the National Nurses in Business Association (NNBA; www.nnbanow.com) as well as state and national associations of coaches and counselors. Additionally, your alma mater and other local schools may offer free or nominal-fee career services. You can also do an online search for "nurses career coach" and look in magazine and newspaper classified ads under "Services Offered." Make sure the person you choose to work with has the expertise and skills you need and is someone you feel comfortable working with. Fees vary so be sure to ask about costs up front.

Mentors, Role Models, and Advisors

If there is someone you know and you have a relationship with, work with, or admire from afar, consider having a brief conversation with them in person or by telephone to discuss career-related issues (email and SM communication are not ideal in this situation). Mentors, role models, and advisors take many forms. They might be doing something you aspire to do and be able to give you advice and support. Perhaps they are successful in their own right and can give insights and information about a particular industry or provide inspiration and encouragement to you. Consider someone who has overcome obstacles or adversity to get where they are and can motivate you to take your career to the next level. Read more about mentoring in chapter 10.

Letting the Universe Work for You

Sometimes a job finds you, rather than you finding a job. You may or may not be looking for a new position when an opportunity presents itself. It may be something you have never done before or even considered doing, yet there are elements of the position or specialty that intrigue and attract you. If this happens to you, at the very least gather more information, go on an interview if you have the opportunity, and take some time to think about what it might mean for you.

Be open to new ideas and opportunities. Sometimes a seemingly random event is the universe's way of lighting your path. One nurse recently said to me, "I've been unlucky in my career. I've been laid off four times in the last 4 years." I suggested that maybe fate was playing a hand and giving her a gentle boot out into the world of unconventional work options. When I suggested this, she admitted that she had always wanted to start her own nursing business but never had the courage to break out on her own. She suddenly saw her misfortune as an opportunity to move in a new direction. There is always more than one door.

Learn to listen to your inner voices and trust your instincts. We often resist that which pulls us or interests us. The philosopher Johann Wolfgang von Goethe said, "As soon as you trust yourself, you will know how to live." If you relax into your life, let down some of your defenses, and push away some of the brambles in your mind, you may see a path that was previously hidden from view. This internal listening and knowing sometimes requires spending quiet time away from the distractions of everyday life, including television, radio, and other electronic devices. The library, a park, a house of worship, a museum, or even a special room of your house can provide such space.

Challenges to Moving Forward

All this talk about stepping out of your comfort zone, creating momentum, expanding your horizons, and moving forward is probably making you a little nervous, right? That's normal. The following are some common obstacles to getting on with your career as well as some practical solutions for getting beyond them.

The Fear Factor

Fear is a powerful force in our lives. Too often, it keeps us from realizing our dreams, developing our full potential, and reaching self-actualization. Moving forward in your career involves making changes and trying new things, and that is scary stuff for most of us. Humans resist change and prefer to maintain the status quo, but no growth occurs without change. That doesn't mean you necessarily have to change jobs; it means you have to step out of your comfort zone and stretch yourself. *Understand that whenever you're making changes or trying something new, fear is automatically part of the equation.* If you didn't feel some degree of fear and anxiety, then you wouldn't be challenging yourself. Even successful people are afraid of making changes, trying new things, and taking their careers to the next level. They have just learned to move forward in spite of that fear.

For some of us, fear becomes a self-imposed barrier that stands between us and our destiny. I once read a quotation that said, "We are like prisoners in a cell where the door is open and the jailer is gone." That quote conjures up an image of the self-imposed imprisonment many of us put ourselves in. We never move forward in our careers because we fear so much; we fear failure and success, the unknown, looking foolish, and not knowing what we're doing.

So how can you better cope with your fears?

- Acknowledge and accept them. Rather than letting fear become an obstacle, learn to bring it along with you as you move forward, knowing that it is part and parcel of stretching yourself. Think of it as growing pains. Mark Twain wrote in *Pudd'nhead Wilson* (1894), "Courage is resistance to fear, mastery of fear—not absence of fear."

- Look for support and encouragement from friends and family and like-minded individuals. As Les Brown, author and motivational speaker, says, "Sometimes you've got to believe in someone else's belief in you until your own belief kicks in." If there's something you want to do, look to those who believe in you or others already doing that thing for support and guidance.

- Face your fears head on. Often, our fear of doing something is much worse than actually doing it. Remember, you only have to do something for the first time once. And, as already mentioned, nurses are highly intelligent individuals and quick learners. We're adaptable, flexible, and versatile. We're capable of much more than we give ourselves credit for.

- Get yourself pumped up and positive. Many fears are based on our feelings of inadequacy and self-doubt. And those feelings become magnified in the face of new challenges and transitions. Shift your focus by reading and listening to motivational materials. Write down positive things people have said about you. Make a list of your past accomplishments. We often think in terms of where we are now and where we still want to go. We forget about how far we've already come. When you focus on the positive, it becomes your reality. It also helps put your fears into perspective.

Excuses, Excuses, Excuses

Instead of making commitments, many of us make excuses. We all have our favorite excuses that we're fond of using to convince ourselves why we can't do something or can't move forward in our lives. Excuses are simply self-made obstacles. Excuses usually take two forms: the "I can't because" excuses and the "I'm waiting for" excuses.

"*I can't because...* I'm too old... I'm too young... I don't have the right experience... I'm not smart enough... I'm too fat... I've been in nursing too long... I've been out of nursing too long... My biorhythms are out of whack... I don't have a college degree... I don't have a high enough degree... I have too many advanced degrees...." The list goes on and on. We have an incredible knack for taking our own circumstances and turning them into convenient, yet unfounded, reasons not to move forward.

"*I'm waiting for...* My kids to finish college... My kids to leave home... My spouse to leave home... My bank account to be bigger... Circumstances to be ideal... My waistline to be smaller... Hell to freeze over...." Many of these may never happen, but we cling steadfastly to them. And if one situation resolves itself, we can easily substitute another excuse to prolong our waiting, thus avoiding growth ad infinitum.

Believe me when I tell you that I have heard every excuse in the book at one time or another and even used some of them myself along the way. In reality, you can do anything you put your mind to. If you make something a priority in your life, you'll find a way to work it out. Every perceived obstacle can be overcome. And if you're waiting for circumstances to be what you envision as ideal in your life, you're setting yourself up for failure since so many other things can happen while you're waiting. You're making an assumption that everything will remain status quo in your life while you wait: your job, your health, your financial situation, your family structure, the economy, and so on. In truth, there will never be a better time than now to move forward, even in a small way.

Indecision

Many of us sit on the fence for a good part of our career trying to decide which direction to move in. We avoid making decisions because we're afraid of living with the consequences of wrong decisions. But not making a decision is a decision in itself; it's a decision to keep things as they are, and there are consequences associated with that, too. The ability to make good career decisions is an important part of moving forward. We are more in control of our lives and careers than most of us want to admit. Anthony Robbins, self-help guru, says, "I believe it's our decisions, not the conditions of our lives, that determine our destiny."

No career decisions are perfect, and none are wrong. There are only different paths to follow and different experiences to have. You have to make career choices based on the best information available to you, where you are right now in your life and career, and where you might be headed. You should make those choices based on your interests, needs, instincts, and the options available to you. Of course you can't always be certain of the outcome when you make a decision. You have to make your choice and move forward with faith.

Often, indecision is masking fear. We say, "I don't know what I want to do," when in reality the truth, or what would be required to make what we want a reality, is too frightening to think about. As mentioned above, some of us fear success as much as we fear failure and worry about how it will change our lives, others' perceptions of us, and our own view of the world. Of course, in some cases, we are simply overwhelmed with the sheer number of choices available and have trouble sorting through them all.

The good news is that once you learn the appropriate steps, good decision-making is something you get better at with practice.

How to facilitate the decision-making process:

- Consider what you want and need based on self-assessment and your current level of career satisfaction and happiness. Is there something you need to change? Something you want to do? Something you'd like to try? Write down what is most important to you and what you're most interested in. Consider possible options and solutions.

- Gather more information. For example, if you're having difficulty deciding on a degree major, request catalogs from nearby colleges, online programs, or both. This will allow you to review the coursework for various majors, the admission requirements, number of credits required, fees involved, and more. All of this is vital information in choosing a school and a major. You can also go the public library and browse through books in the reference section such as *The College Blue Book* (be sure it's a current edition), which list schools and majors such as "Health Care," "Business," "Social Sciences," and so forth. You may discover a degree program you weren't aware of. Ask the librarian or use the Internet to help you find these and other related resources.

- If you're considering changing specialties, use the steps mentioned previously under "Explore Career Options." If you're considering starting a business, get to the public library or the Internet and see what's required to start a business in your state, including any special requirements for the specific type of business you're considering. You can't make an informed decision until you have all the facts.

- Talk to people in the know. Get in touch with people who have done something similar, who are working in a field you're considering, or have pursued a degree you're thinking about. They can give you a unique perspective and inside information that you may not have thought about. People have different opinions and experiences, so talk to several people and accept that you may have to sort through the advice and information to find what you need.

- Write about it. Writing can be very therapeutic and can help clarify your thoughts. Whether you put pen to paper or fingers to keyboard, the very act of writing down what's on your mind, including your questions and your dilemmas, can help you work toward decisions and solutions.

- Talk it over with a friend or trusted colleague. When you have an important decision to make, talking it out can be very helpful. Saying things out loud gives you a different perspective than thinking about it or even writing about it. You can also get feedback and input from the person with whom you're speaking.

- Go with your gut. When all is said and done, only you can make a decision that's right for you. Do all of the above and then listen to your heart. Once you make a decision, make a commitment to make it work. Then take action to make it happen, even a small step in the right direction.

Risk Avoidance

Whether or not you consider yourself a risk taker, you take risks every day in the course of your life and work. There are risks associated with everything you do. You can't avoid them; you can only minimize them. How? By getting as much information as you can, talking to experienced, knowledgeable people, doing some soul-searching, and considering what you hope to gain from any situation. Why take risks at all? Because they create opportunities, vitality, and growth in your career, and are a necessary step to reaching your full potential.

When considering taking any career risks, whether changing special-ties, quitting your job, taking a higher level position, or taking on more responsibility, ask yourself, "What's the worst that can happen if I do this?" Possible answers include: "I could hate it; I could not do as well at it as I was hoping; I might not get along with the people; I might miss my current coworkers." Then also ask yourself "What's the best that could happen if I do this?" Possible answers include: "I could love It; I could excel at it; it could lead to other things; I can grow and utilize more of my potential and talents; I could make some great contacts and some new friends."

You've heard the expression, "Nothing ventured, nothing gained." Although the lure of the comfort zone is strong, there is no progress without some intelligent risk taking.

Other benefits can only be realized once you take the risks. Remember the job I took with the company that did medical exams for insurance compa-nies? I took a significant risk on many levels in accepting that position. I left the relative security of a cushy job with a good company to do some-thing totally different. I also took a significant pay cut to work there. I knew that the job offered avenues for learning and the type of low-key environ-ment and work schedule I was looking for. I couldn't possibly have known that a brand new system of health care reimbursement (the DRG system) would be implemented while I was working there and that I would have an opportunity to be trained in its use. Yet that turned out to be one of the biggest opportunities of my career, leading me to a position in a hospital where I first began to form my vision of becoming a public speaker and a career coach. Was I simply lucky? Luck had nothing to do with it. This is the type of thing that happens when you get yourself out there, move forward in your career, make decisions, and take calculated career risks.

There is no failure, only different lessons to learn. Concentrate less on the outcome and more on the experience. Joy and benefits come from just doing and trying. Not everything is about outcomes. Focus on the journey. It is all part of the process of learning, growing, and moving forward.

MY HERO

Each of us has our heroes in nursing: people we admire for their clinical skills, compassionate caring nature, levelheadedness, what they've done with their careers, or a combination of those aspects. One of my nursing heroes is a woman named Rosemary. We worked together years ago and stayed in touch over the years. She is one of the most competent and caring nurses I have ever known. Her intelligence, clear thinking, uncompromising values, nursing intuition, and commitment to her profession have always impressed me. I have learned much from her over the years. She is one of the quiet heroes of our profession.

I recently asked her why she became a nurse. I was interested to know what brought her to where she is today. Her answer shocked me. "I almost *didn't* become a nurse after a high school guidance counselor told me I wasn't smart enough," she said. "I knew I wanted to be a nurse from the fifth or sixth grade. I had visited a Veteran's Administration hospital with a Girl Scout troop one Christmas holiday. There were a lot of very sick people there. All of my friends couldn't wait to leave, yet I wanted to stay. I was somehow drawn to the place, the patients. I almost felt as if I belonged there. I later wrote a school paper about the nursing profession and got an A on it, and I didn't get too many As back then!

"So when it became time to plot my future, I not only knew exactly what I wanted to do, but I even knew what nursing school I wanted to go to. When I relayed this to my guidance counselor, she uttered those words I will never forget: 'You're not smart enough to be a nurse.' To add salt to the wound she added, 'Besides, you would never get accepted into that school.' I was devastated. I took her at her word and dropped my plans to follow my dream. Instead, I took an office job out of high school and was absolutely miserable.

"My mother knew how unhappy I was and in an effort to help, mentioned an LPN [licensed practical nurse] program being offered in our area to county residents. My guidance counselor's words rang in my head, and I thought to myself, 'But I'm not smart enough.' I decided to give it a shot anyway. As it turns out, I got a great education and happily worked as an LPN for 5 years. I then enrolled in a university program to become an RN/BSN. I was on a roll."

Over the years, Rosemary worked as a staff nurse in critical care, then as the charge nurse on a telemetry unit, manager in cardiac rehab, part of the staff education team, utilization review nurse, head nurse in oncology, and a member of the float pool. She eventually became a certified diabetic educator.

Rosemary worked all of her RN career to that point in the same hospital. That is where I came to know her. I used to tease her that she should

(continued)

receive an award for having the most positions within the shortest amount of time at one place of employment. She had eight different positions in 18 years. She said, "I had so many interests and so many opportunities. I was always learning something new and was open to new challenges and experiences." Years later, Rosemary decided to go to graduate school and become a nurse practitioner. Today, she has a collaborative arrangement with several physicians in a busy cardiology practice.

Rosemary's advice to others: "Be true to yourself. Don't ever let someone else tell you what you should or shouldn't do with your life. And don't let anyone else shatter your dreams. If you want to do something badly enough, there is always a way to do it. Go for it!"

Chapter 4

Looking for Your Next Job

Whether in the job market by choice or necessity, job-finding basics are the same. And while most people usually look for employment in print or online ads, there are many other—often more effective—ways to find and land a good job.

Networking—Your Best Choice

In chapters 2 and 3, we discussed networking to explore career options, to obtain information about specialties, and to stay connected. Networking is also one of the best and most effective ways to find and get a good job. Estimates are that 50%–90% of all jobs are found through networking or word of mouth. Personal contacts and connections are your best source when in the job market. Does that mean you have to personally know someone in a particular specialty or who works for a company to get in? Not at all. Chances are that you know someone, who knows someone else, who knows someone else who can put you in touch with someone who knows someone who can help you. The more people you talk to, the larger your network becomes and the greater the chance you have these connections.

You may have heard someone say, "I got this job through dumb luck. It just fell into my lap. I was talking to my neighbor when he mentioned his company was looking for a nurse." That's not dumb luck, that's networking. Sometimes you may initiate the networking contacts; other times contacts may come to you. The process works rather well, which is why you should always stay connected and visible. It's whom you know, and who knows you, that will contribute to your success.

Networking with the objective of finding job opportunities involves launching a targeted campaign to connect with those you already know, to make new strategic contacts, and to cultivate ongoing relationships with old and new contacts. It also involves becoming visible through professional and social channels. Networking will help you uncover unadvertised or "hidden" jobs, provide introductions to decision-makers, and provide insider information on an industry, positions, companies, salaries, and other employment information.

So how can you use networking in the job search process? Let's count the ways.

First Things First

Networking with the objective of job seeking uses strategies that go beyond networking to merely stay connected. A business card is one fundamental to any networking situation, but it is particularly vital when looking for a job (see chapter 10). Even if you're currently employed and have a business card related to your present position, you should have a card with personal contact information just for networking. This way people can contact you outside of work and long after you've left your current employment. Remember to carry those cards with you wherever you go because you never know whom you'll meet.

Who Ya Gonna Call?

The easiest way to launch your networking campaign is to get on the telephone and start contacting former coworkers and supervisors, nursing instructors and colleagues, physicians, and others who know you. Don't limit your contacts to health care workers since everyone has connections in different industries. The power of networking is that people know people who know other people, in all walks of life.

If you haven't spoken to any of your contacts in a while, take a minute to catch up. Ask them how they're doing and what they've been up to. Let them know you're alive and well and in the job market. If there's something specific you're interested in, say so. For example, "I'm looking to get into research working for a pharmaceutical company," or "I'm looking to transition into labor and delivery."

If you don't know exactly what you want to do, you can let people know that you're in the market for "something different." Of course, the more specific you are, the better. If you're not sure what you're looking for, then at least narrow your search. For instance, you might tell people that you do or don't want to work in a hospital, are looking for something you can do from home, or prefer a job largely done on the computer. You can also say something general, such as "I'm looking to do something different from what I've done in the past. I'd ideally like to work from home using my computer. Please keep your ears open for me. I'm exploring my options." Because you want to continuously expand your network, always add, "Do you know anyone else I might be able to speak with?" If they give you a contact, add, "May I say that you referred me?" Getting referrals is important because a mutual connection with someone you're contacting is better than contacting someone "cold." Use that connection when calling and writing by indicating who referred you or suggested the contact.

If you know what you want to do and happen to know someone who works in that industry, start there. For example, if you want to break into the pharmaceutical industry, you should contact anyone you know who is associated in any way with that industry, regardless of their position. Let them know of your interest and ask for their help in achieving your goal. You might say something like, "I'm very interested in exploring a career in pharmaceutical research. I was hoping you could refer me to someone in the research department at your company. I'd also appreciate any advice you can give me about breaking into the field. I value your opinion."

As another example, if you wanted to change specialties and get into labor and delivery, it would make sense to talk to anyone you know who works in that specialty, regardless of their employer or location. How can acquaintances who work at other hospitals in other cities possibly help you get a position in a local hospital? They may be connected through professional associations, through former employers, and even through friends and family.

One of my favorite networking stories comes from a nurse who seized an opportunity on the very day she was attending one of my seminars. We were in a large city and the group was on lunch break. During that time, this nurse was walking outside and saw a large group of people walking out of another hotel, all carrying canvas bags emblazoned with the logo of a well-known pharmaceutical company. Having just heard my spiel about networking, she decided to approach one member of the group. She said, "I couldn't help noticing your tote bags. I'm a nurse and have always been interested in working in your industry." The woman she approached was also a nurse, and she said, "I'd be happy to help you, do you have a business card?" (Get those cards made!) She did not, but asked for the person's card and said she would contact her later. Opportunities are everywhere, if you just look for them.

Once you've made connections, stay in touch with them and keep them posted on your progress. Invite them to connect on LinkedIn (LI) and follow them on Twitter. An email follow-up is OK for networking encounters, especially a short note right after the meeting or phone call. But I encourage you to send a handwritten follow-up note (if your penmanship

THE POWER OF NETWORKING

A nurse who had just relocated to my area recently contacted me. She wanted to work in a dermatology office in her new location. She heard me talk about the value of networking in job hunting and called me for advice. She knew people who worked in dermatology in her old location, but she didn't know anyone here or how to start her networking. I told her to begin with connections from her former locale by letting them know where she was and what she was looking for. Perplexed, she responded, "But I want to work in this state, not in the one I just left." I explained that people have connections all over the country. Professional people join national associations and attend conventions. They probably have associates who have relocated themselves. I emphasized that networking does not have to be done only with people who directly work for a company or facility for which you wish to work or even live in the same state. Networking knows no geographic boundaries. Just because people live elsewhere doesn't mean they don't have contacts and connections in other areas.

Remember, you shouldn't limit networking efforts to those who work in a particular specialty or even to those in health care. You never know who has a brother, cousin, or neighbor who works in the industry or for a company in which you want to be employed. The power of networking is far-reaching, so you should cast your net widely.

Networking at Its Best

I once received a phone call from a nurse who had attended my Career Alternatives for Nurses seminar. She was very excited and wanted to tell me about a positive networking experience.

"The weekend after your seminar, I attended a block party in my neighborhood. I remembered what you said about 'getting the word out' and decided to let those I spoke with know I was in the job market. I was talking to a man I knew through church. I'd heard he was an accountant, but I didn't know much else about him. In the course of conversation, I mentioned that I wanted to get into pharmaceutical research. He said, 'Really? I work for XXX Pharmaceutical Company. I could probably refer you to someone in the research department there.' I was dumbstruck for a moment, but then said, 'You're kidding. I thought you were an accountant.' He said, 'I am an accountant, but I happen to work for XXX.'" A week later this nurse had a job interview with this company and a month later, a job offer. She was astonished at how a casual conversation at a social function with someone she didn't know well could lead to such an incredible opportunity. That's networking at its best!

is legible and neat) after a meeting or a phone call. People appreciate the effort and it will make you more memorable. Include your business card in the note, even if you previously gave one. Having business cards in your contacts' hands or on their desks is a good way to keep you fresh in their mind. It's also necessary if they want or need to get in touch with you or refer someone to you. Any correspondence you have with your connections, including email, should always include contact information. Don't make anyone work to get in touch with you. Keep an online or hard copy file of your contacts, when and where you met them, and any advice or referrals they gave you. Stay organized and remember the origins of your leads so you can update and thank the right person afterward.

Get Yourself Out There and Be Visible

While online connections are important, your job-hunting campaign should include getting out on a regular basis to career fairs, professional association meetings, nursing conventions, and conferences. In addition to nursing and health care career fairs, go to industry-specific career fairs, such as those run for the pharmaceutical and information technology industries. Consider also attending general career fairs, where all types of positions are made available, as there are invariably numerous health care facilities and companies exhibiting there. These events are advertised in trade publications and in such mainstream media as newspapers, radio, and the Internet. Opportunities are everywhere.

You should also attend open houses, open interviews, and recruitment events offered by prospective employers, even if you're not sure what they have to offer or whether you even want to work for them. Attending such events is a great way to learn more and make great contacts. You just never know where the spark, idea, connection, or opportunity will come from! Remember that face-to-face networking is most effective. Plus, it helps keep your social skills sharp, as they can get rusty when you don't use them regularly!

TIME WELL SPENT

I recently heard from a nurse who told me she always thought attending career fairs was a waste of time. After reading one of my articles, she decided to get out to a nursing career fair in her area. Later she informed me that she had found her dream job there, an entry-level position doing a specialized type of case management, working for a private review company. Anything can happen when you get yourself out there.

Informational Interviewing

An informational interview, also known as an information-gathering interview, is a more formal type of networking. It involves a formal interview, that is, talking in a structured way to someone who works in a specialty you are interested in or for a company you wish to work for.

Informational interviewing is an effective way to learn more about a particular specialty and position. It's a good way to get inside information about a company or industry, too. It can yield advice about breaking into that industry or specialty as well as provide specific contacts. Informational interviewing may give you a foot in the door as well as indirect access to hidden jobs in the company, referrals to jobs at other companies, a straight job offer, or a decision-maker in a company and other influential people in a specialty. Since the major objective of an informational interview is to get information, advice, and additional contacts, you should not ask for a job. However, if one is offered, that would be a bonus. Informational

EIGHT STEPS TO MAXIMIZE YOUR TIME AT A CAREER FAIR OR CONVENTION

1. **Dress to Impress**: Make a good impression even if you're not actively looking for a job. Stand out from the crowd as a polished professional. Dress as you would for an interview (wear a suit or your best outfit—see chapter 8). You'll make some of your most important professional contacts at these events and you want to look sharp.

2. **Determine Your Objective**: Consider what you want to accomplish while there. Are you seeking a job offer or exploring career options? Do you want to gather information about graduate schools? Are you seeking a personal connection with an editor or publisher who may be there? Think about what is most important to you and how your time will be best spent.

3. **Scan the Exhibitors' List**: Most events provide a list of exhibitors along with their location in the exhibit hall. Scan the list for those you'd most like to connect with and visit those booths first. This will ensure that you have sufficient time to make your most important contacts. You can use your remaining time to browse the exhibitor floor or visit secondary targets.

4. **Make Personal Contacts**: Approach selected exhibitors with direct eye contact and a smile. Introduce yourself with a full, firm handshake. Ask about the company or facility they represent and inquire about what opportunities exist there for nurses, if appropriate. Remember, these events are not just for job hunting. You're gathering information and making important contacts.

5. **Carry Business Cards**: Personal or work-related business cards are a great way to exchange contact information and are essential for professional networking. See chapter 10 for the whys and how-tos of creating and carrying cards. Some nurses also carry preprinted address labels to save time when adding their contact information to the mailing list of selected vendors.

6. **Follow Up**: Always reinforce your initial contacts by sending a note or making a phone call. Let them know you enjoyed meeting them and follow up on anything discussed. Because this is not an interview follow-up, it would be appropriate to send an email or handwritten follow-up note here. Connect on LI and Twitter too. Be sure to ask for the card of anyone you wish to stay in touch with or may want to contact at a later date. To jog your memory later, jot down on the back of their cards where and when you met them and any important issues discussed.

(continued)

7. **Bring Your Résumé:** Regardless of your purpose in attending, it is always wise to bring updated copies of your résumé to these events. You never know what might come up or who will request a copy. Even if you're happily employed, you may discover an opportunity to do some consulting on the side, some writing or teaching, or even learn of a career opportunity that you never considered. It's best to be prepared. Carry them unfolded in a portfolio.

8. **Act Professional:** While it's OK to avail yourself of some of the free samples offered by vendors, such as pens and candy, it is appropriate to first make eye contact and greet the vendor before taking anything. It's also polite to ask first, too, since everything on the table is not necessarily a free sample. Some vendors have had books and CDs that were for sale as well as their own personal pens and mugs taken by overzealous attendees. Likewise, it is appropriate to take one of something that is offered for free, not a handful, unless otherwise indicated.

interviewing is a valuable networking tool even if you are not yet actively seeking employment and just exploring options.

Here's how it works: Make a list of people you'd like to talk to, and not necessarily people you already know. You could list people who work in a particular industry, who are doing something you'd like to do, people you admire, or people you'd like to work for. The list might include officers of a related professional association at state, national, or local levels. For example, if you were considering getting into infection control, you might arrange an informational interview with the state chapter president of the Association for Professionals in Infection Control and Epidemiology (APIC).

While informational interviewing can be done by telephone, or email if necessary, an in-person meeting is always preferable and should be your objective. That is because, as previously mentioned, face-to-face networking is more powerful than any other method. The opportunity to meet, shake hands, and interact with someone up close and personal is the most effective approach you can use. Of course, if the person you wish to speak with is not geographically near you, a telephone interview will suffice. When arranging for a telephone interview, ask the person if they prefer to get the questions ahead of time by email.

Make initial contact with each person by telephone or with a letter of introduction (see example at end of chapter). Email can be used for an initial contact to set up an appointment to speak further. However, a hard copy letter in the mail, such as the one mentioned above, is preferable because it is more formal and allows you to carefully state your interest and intent. A formal letter should always be followed up by a phone call.

Note: It is not advisable to send important personal communication via social media (SM) such as Facebook or LI as many people do not read these messages.

If making an initial contact by phone, be prepared with what you want to say. Start with a brief introduction and then be sure the person is free to speak with you briefly. Say something like, "Hi Ms. Arnold. My name is Carol Jenkins, and I'm a registered nurse interested in learning more about psychiatric nursing. Do you have a moment to speak with me?" If Ms. Arnold says yes, then you can continue with something like, "I'd love the opportunity to meet with you in person to ask you some questions about psychiatric nursing and to learn more about you and how you got into your current position." If Ms. Arnold were to say, "Are you looking for a job? Because we don't have any openings right now," you might respond by saying, "That's not why I'm calling you. I'm looking for some information and advice."

Ms. Arnold might then respond by saying, "Well, can't we do this over the phone?" Since your objective is to get an in-person meeting, you might say something like, "We could, but I've prepared a résumé and would appreciate it if you could look it over and give me some advice." If Ms. Arnold says, "Well why don't you email it to me?" you could counter with, "I could do that, but I know that the overall appearance of my résumé, as well as the content, is important. Besides, I would be thrilled to meet you face-to-face and have an opportunity to speak to you in person." That approach is hard to resist. In other words, be persuasive and overcome objections to get that meeting. You may have to sell the idea to some people, but believe me, it will pay off for you.

In spite of your best efforts, there will always be some people who can't or won't agree to meet you in person. Perhaps they are overloaded with work, have personal challenges, or are trying to meet a deadline. In that case, try to at least get some phone time from them. Be prepared with your questions whenever you call someone in case they say, "Gee I'd love to meet with you, but we're being surveyed in a month, and I just can't spare the time. However, I have a few moments now if you want to ask me some questions," or, "If you send me your questions by email, I'll answer them when I have a few moments." Take whatever you can get. On the rare occasion that you encounter someone who seems put off by your request, thank them for their time, wish them a good day, and move on to your next contact.

Always set a specific timeframe for the meeting and stick to it. For example, you might say or write, "I'll only take 20 minutes of your time." If they say, "I can only give you 15 minutes," take it.

For an in-person informational interview, dress as you would for a job interview (see chapter 8). Bring a small notebook or tablet with you and have your questions written down so you don't forget anything. It is perfectly appropriate to take handwritten notes during the interview, but typing on an electronic device can be distracting. Just don't write nonstop since you want to have eye contact and some personal interaction with the individual. You want them to get to know you, too.

Questions to ask include:

- How did you get started in the specialty?
- What do you like most and least about your job?
- What is the job outlook for the next five years in this specialty or industry?
- Can you describe a typical day?
- Are there any industry trends I should know about?
- What professional associations do you or others in this specialty belong to?
- What are typical salary ranges in this specialty for entry-level, mid-level, and advanced positions?
- What advice do you have for someone interested in breaking into the specialty?
- How do you see someone like me fitting into this specialty?
- Do you know anyone else I can talk to? If yes: Can I say that you referred me?

After the interview, whether it was by phone, email, or in-person, send a thank-you note. Thank the person for their time, sage advice, and insights. Then stay in periodic touch with them. If they gave you a lead or referral, follow up with them and let them know how you made out. Keep them posted on your progress and do let them know when you find a position. A networking thank-you note can be handwritten or typed. Since an informational interview is a more formal type of networking, I recommend sending a typed letter on good stationery, but do use your judgment here. Whether handwritten or typed, the important thing is that you send the note. It's also OK to send a short email or text message the day of the meeting to say thanks. But this would be in addition to the typed or written note sent via post mail.

Common Misgivings

You may be hesitant to approach people with this method because you are not accustomed to asking for help. But asking for help is not a sign of weakness, as many fear. Rather, it is a sign that you are intelligent, assertive, and humble enough to know you have a lot to learn.

You might also be asking yourself, "Why would a total stranger want to help me?" Contrary to what you might believe, most people have a natural instinct to want to help others. Most people are sincerely glad to be of assistance if approached in the right manner. When you approach someone with courtesy and respect, show interest in them and their specialty, and exhibit enthusiasm, you will be surprised at how total strangers will bend over backward to help you. Why? For some people it is an ego boost to be sought out for advice. Others will identify with your situation and remember when they were first getting started. The latter is certainly true for me; I am always happy to give advice or guidance to someone who asks. Many others helped me along the way, and I am only too happy to pass that on. Most people feel that way. That's what makes the world go round.

Networking is unquestionably the best and most effective way to find a job. But a successful job search campaign will employ many different strategies for maximum benefit, such as those in the following sections.

The Classified Ads

The want ads, also known as the classified ads, are the most commonly used yet least effective method of finding jobs. Estimates are that only 5%–10% of all available jobs ever get into the classifieds, whether in print or online. That's probably surprising to those of you who rely so heavily on them. The higher the level and more desirable the position, the less likely it is to appear in the classifieds. Why? These positions are filled primarily through word of mouth and other means, which we'll discuss in a moment.

However, don't ignore these ads because they can lead to some interesting positions. They can also open doors of opportunity and uncover hidden jobs, as they did for me early in my career. There are multiple sources of classified ads so be sure to explore them all. Here are the most common ones:

Nursing and health care magazines. Targeted classifieds, such as those found in industry journals, can yield some good information. In addition to general nursing magazines, be sure to check the classified ads in nursing and health care publications specifically geared to managers and administrators. Also, use specialty journals for related classified ads. For example, if you were looking for a position in occupational health nursing, you'd want to check out the ads in *Workplace Health & Safety*, the official publication of the American Association of Occupational Health Nurses (AAOHN). You can find these publications in the health sciences library of a local hospital or the periodical section of a college library that offers degrees in nursing or health care.

Public newspapers. Be sure to check the large circulation newspapers in your area, both print and online, including those of nearby big cities. For example, if you want to work in New Jersey, you would naturally check the New Jersey newspapers. However, the *New York Times* and the *Philadelphia Inquirer* also carry ads for positions in New Jersey because of their proximity. Don't just look in the health care section of the ads, either. Some companies will post relevant positions under headings, such as "Sales," "Medical," "Computers," and others. Be sure to look in the large display ads in the front of the classified section too.

The Internet. The Internet is a vast source of classified ads. You'll find job postings on career-related web sites, professional association web sites, company and facility web sites, and employment and nursing agency web sites. Many newspapers and magazines also post ads both in print and on their web site.

Even though the Internet seems like a convenient and abundant source of ads, keep in mind that these are still classified ads and as such only represent a small percentage of all available jobs. We'll discuss posting your résumé online in chapter 6. Again, that may yield you some job prospects, but your time could be better spent by getting on the telephone and networking or getting out to some career events or conventions. Relying solely on your paperwork (e.g., résumés and cover letters) to sell you is one of the toughest ways to find and get a job.

Keep in mind that classifieds are open jobs. That means they are publicly advertised, so often there are many applicants representing a lot of competition for the same job. We'll discuss cover letters in chapter 6 as a way to make yourself stand out. Many more effective and direct approaches can be used to uncover hidden jobs, such as making direct contact with prospective employers. The following are a few ways to do that.

ATTITUDE IS EVERYTHING

Read classified ads with a grain of salt. Often the specifications in an ad are not set in stone and are more flexible than the average reader realizes. Ads that state certain credentials or experience are "desirable," "preferred," "ideal," or "a plus" only mean that it would be nice but isn't necessary. Even if an ad says that something is "required," that point is often more negotiable than you might think. If you see an ad that appeals to you, you should give it your best shot.

Several years ago, I met a young nurse who had recently graduated from an associate's degree program. She was interested in research and applied for a part-time research position she saw advertised at a local university. The ad stated that all candidates must have at least three years of clinical experience and a minimum of a bachelor's degree, master's degree preferred. This recently graduated nurse did not meet any of those specifications but applied for the job anyway. She was offered the job and happily accepted.

How could this happen? Because when all is said and done, prospective employers are looking to hire a personality, not just a body to fill a slot. This young nurse was personable, professional, and enthusiastic about research. Attitude is everything.

Direct Mail Campaign

A direct mail campaign involves sending a post mail letter of introduction and interest to a specific company or person you'd like to work for (see example at end of chapter). It is a targeted job search technique used to uncover unadvertised jobs in a particular company or industry and to gain access to industry leaders. The approach is somewhat different from requesting an informational interview in that you are directly asking for a job. For example, if you wished to work for a health care information technology (HIT) company or wanted to break into quality improvement (QI), you would target certain companies and facilities that might offer these positions. You would then identify a decision-maker for the specific department or division you'd like to work for—that is, someone who has the authority to actually hire you. This might be a department director, a division manager, a vice president, a regional director, or the like.

Let's say you wanted to get into QI. You would target health care facilities, insurance companies, and private review companies that offer such positions. You would then identify a decision-maker in a related department, such as the director of QI, by asking around, looking at company web sites, doing a general Internet search, searching on LI, or calling the company or department directly. You might contact a local hospital and say, "Could you please give me the name and title of the person in charge of the quality improvement department?" Hopefully, the person answering the phone will have that information or will transfer you to someone who does. Be sure to get the exact spelling of the person's name, their exact title, and any credentials if applicable (e.g., RN, PhD, etc.). If you are asked why you want the information, you can simply say, "I want to send them something in the mail," which is true. Do not say you are looking for a job because you will be put through to human resources (HR) instead.

If you've decided you wanted to work for a particular product company, such as one that makes computer software for nurses or one that makes heart monitors or respirators, decide what capacity you want to work in and then identify the appropriate decision-maker. For example, are you interested in sales and marketing or training and development, or do you wish to work as a clinical consultant? If you're not sure, do some informational interviewing first.

Marketing Letter Basics

Marketing letters for your direct mail campaign should be sent to those who have direct authority to hire you, not to HR. That is because any HR department receives dozens and sometimes hundreds of résumés each day for a wide variety of positions. It may take time for the clerical staff to sort and screen those résumés and see that they get to the right person. Not only do you have additional people scrutinizing your résumé, but the more people who handle it, the more likely it is to get lost or misrouted. With the direct mail approach, you are bypassing the HR department and going directly to the decision-maker.

There are two schools of thought on whether or not to include your résumé with a marketing letter. On the one hand, if a résumé falls out of the envelope, the correspondence may look too much like a job application and the receiver may automatically pass it on to HR for processing without reading the letter. Therefore, if there is no résumé enclosed, you may increase the likelihood of your letter being read and considered. It can serve to whet the reader's appetite and leave them wanting more information. Of course, you should highlight your relevant experience in your letter. On the other hand, if a prospective employer is intrigued by your letter, they may be frustrated or annoyed that you have not included your résumé with additional details about your background. Consider both perspectives when deciding whether to send a résumé or not on the initial contact.

Every marketing letter must be followed up with a phone call. Don't even bother to send them out if you don't intend to do this. Remember, you're asking the prospective employer for a job, so you need to remain proactive in the situation. Don't just throw the ball into their lap and expect them to act on it. You want something from them and have to pursue it. End every marketing letter with a statement indicating that you will call in a week as a follow-up (see example at end of chapter).

When you make the follow-up call, several things may happen. You might get a gatekeeper, such as a receptionist or staff member. In a very assertive voice say something like, "Hi. Carol Roberts calling for Janet Fredericks. Is she in?" If you are asked, "Is she expecting your call?" You would say, "Yes," because you had stated you would call in your letter. If asked what this is in reference to, you can state that it is a follow-up to some correspondence.

If Ms. Fredericks is not in or available, rather than automatically leaving a message, ask, "When is a good time to reach her?" Don't leave a message right away expecting her to call you back. Remember what I said about staying proactive in the situation? Determine another time to call and try again. Likewise, if you keep getting voice mail or an answering machine, don't leave a message right away. Keep calling back on different days and times in an effort to reach her. Try calling before 9 AM and after 5 PM. Many managers and directors are in early and stay late. If the regular office staff is not there, managers and directors will often answer their own telephone.

If you call repeatedly and can't get through to the person you want to speak to, leave a message and state a specific day and time you will call back. For example, you might say, "This is Carol Roberts calling. I sent you a letter last week about my interest in working for you. I've been trying to reach you all week without success. I know you are very busy, so I will try you again this Thursday at 4 PM. If you care to speak with me in the interim, I can be reached at [phone number]." Speak slowly, clearly, and distinctly.

Sound assertive and upbeat. Leaving a message indicating a specific day and time for a callback demonstrates a seriousness of purpose on your part and the recipient is more inclined to take your call or leave a message for you. Of course you do have to call back when you said you would, or you blow your credibility.

If you are unsuccessful reaching the person you wish to speak to by phone, try connecting via SM, indicating that you have been trying to reach them by phone. It's another tool to use but should not be your primary source of initial contact.

Once you reach Ms. Fredericks, introduce yourself briefly and refresh her memory as to who you are. You might say, "Hi, Ms. Fredericks. My name is Carol Roberts. I'm the critical care nurse who wrote to you last week, telling you how much I'd like to work for you. Do you have a moment to speak with me?" If she says, "Yes," be ready with a short statement requesting a meeting with her to further discuss your mutual interests. Then stop talking and let her respond. If she says there are no openings now but she'll keep you in mind, say, "I appreciate that. In the meantime, I'd love to meet you and learn more about you and how you got started in this field. I'd also be grateful if you could look over my résumé and give me a few tips on breaking into this field." In other words, you should not let a great opportunity to connect with this person slip through your fingers just because there are no jobs available. Even if no job is available, they may be able to help you in other ways. Go back to the steps for setting up and conducting an informational interview and take it from there.

Marketing letters can be particularly useful when trying to break into a new specialty or industry and as an adjunct to other job finding methods. Do keep in mind that one-on-one networking is still your best approach in all situations. Now let's look at some methods for getting a third party involved in your job search.

Getting Some Help

There are a number of different types of firms and agencies that match job seekers with employers. Although the term "recruiter" is used in many different settings, there is a difference between the types of agencies they work for and the types of positions and companies they work with. Here are several different categories of organizations and individuals you might seek out to assist you in the job search process.

Professional Recruiters

These individuals, commonly referred to as professional recruiters, head-hunters, and search consultants, search for qualified people to fill specific job openings for client companies. The firm they own or work for is known as a search firm. You might use this type of firm to find a management, administrative, or education position. You might also use this type of firm to find a nontraditional position, such as one in nursing informatics, health care sales and marketing, QI, medical writing, case management, and so on. You would generally not use this type of firm to find a direct patient care position at the staff nurse level.

Here's how professional recruiters work: Their primary client, the one who pays them, is a company or facility that has a professional position that needs to be filled. The recruiter contracts with that company to find quali-fied individuals based on the client's specifications. The recruiter will then scout around for candidates, screen them, and assemble one or more indi-viduals to send to an interview with the client.

Professional recruiters locate candidates primarily by putting the word out to their network. However, you may receive a phone call from recruiters who are looking for a particular type of candidate. I have heard nurses say, "How did they get my name?" or, "How did they find me?" Professional recruiters will sometimes call all area hospitals or health care facilities to speak with nurses in similar positions to those they are working on. If you post your résumé online or have a LinkedIn profile, you may also receive communication from professional recruiters. They may occasionally post a "blind" ad for the position in a newspaper or online looking for quali-fied candidates. A blind ad is one in which no company name appears. A recruiter's ad might read something like, "RN with management experi-ence needed for facility director's position with large metropolitan hospital. Salary range 80K to 90K [$80,000–$90,000]." At the bottom of the ad it may say, "Qualified candidates contact the Henderson Agency," although in some cases, there may only be a PO box or email address.

A recruiter will screen potential candidates by phone and possibly in person if the recruiter and candidate are geographically near one another. Once the candidate is deemed qualified, the recruiter will set up an inter-view for the candidate with the client. The recruiter becomes a go-between for the prospective employer and the job candidate. This means that the job candidate communicates primarily with the recruiter before and after interviews unless otherwise specified.

There are a number of advantages to working with professional recruiters. These recruiters often have access to hidden jobs: those that are not publicly advertised. A recruiter has in-depth knowledge of what their client is looking for and will likely share that information with you. This information can be very helpful during the interview process. A recruiter will usually coach you in the interview process and may even role-play with you to help you deal with challenging questions or potential objections. They may critique your résumé. Additionally, a recruiter will often negotiate salary and benefits for you with the client so you do not have to be directly involved with the company. Just like real estate agents, recruiters are skilled negotiators and can help to seal the deal.

Early in my career, I met a woman who was a recruiter of sales and marketing professionals. She was working on several related positions in the health care industry, and she encouraged me to talk to her further. I wasn't sure that health care sales and marketing was the right direction for me but decided to see how things went. The recruiter sent me on an interview for a company that manufactures respirators. She critiqued my résumé, coached me on what to wear and how to act, and even gave me tips on probable questions I would be asked and how to answer them. This was a great help since I had never been to a corporate interview before. The interview went well, and I was asked back for a second interview, but I decided not to pursue it further. However, it was a great learning experience for me, and I sharpened my interview skills in the process.

After you've been on an interview, the prospective employer will give the recruiter some feedback. The recruiter will likely share that information with you. This can be very helpful in the event of a subsequent interview or in the process of perfecting your self-presentation skills. You'll have a good idea of where you stand and what you need to do to move forward. Remember, the recruiter is motivated to help you get the job. Recruiters don't make any money unless they successfully place someone in a position (more on that in a moment). Another advantage to working with recruiters is that you can get some great interview experience whether you take a job through them or not.

You may be wondering why a company would choose to work with a recruiter rather than fill the position themselves. There are several possible reasons. A company may want to conduct a discreet job search. That is, they may not want the position to be publicly advertised for a variety of reasons. They may not want their competitors to know of the opening, or they may not want their own staff to know of the opening. In some cases, a company simply doesn't want to go through the hassle of advertising for a position, screening candidates, and so forth. They leave that up to the professional recruiter who will just be sending them prescreened candidates for interviews.

Some additional things to know about working with professional recruiters:

Most professional recruiters specialize. They either work within a particular industry or with a particular type of position. For example, some recruiters work exclusively with sales and marketing positions, including health care sales and marketing. Other recruiters work primarily with nursing management positions or health care management in general, both in and out of the hospital. Some recruiters work exclusively with the pharmaceutical industry, information technology industry, or managed care industry.

You are not obligated to take any job you interview for when you work with a recruiter. Of course you should be earnest in your interest and pursuit, but if a job is not right for you, you can say so. It would not be ethical to then directly approach that company about employment for that same position in an effort to circumvent the recruiter. Nor would it be ethical to refer a friend to that company for the same position. For that reason, a recruiter may not reveal the name of a client until they are ready to send you on an interview. But remember that recruiters are not being cagey or secretive; they are simply protecting their own interests.

The recruiter makes money by receiving a fee from the client—the employer—once the recruiter has successfully placed a candidate in that position. A recruiter's fee is usually a percentage of the salary the candidate is hired at, although sometimes other arrangements are made. For example, if you were hired at $80,000, and the recruiter had an agreement with the client to place a candidate for 20% of the annual starting salary, the recruiter would receive a fee of $16,000 for the service. Some recruiters are paid a retainer fee, rather than a commission, for the service they provide.

You, the candidate, should never pay a fee to a professional recruiter. In fact, this is actually illegal in many cases. You should also be wary of a recruiter that offers additional services for a fee, such as résumé writing, interview coaching, or career counseling. Many recruiters offer these services at no cost to job candidates.

Frequently Asked Questions

Q: *How can I locate a professional recruiter?*

A: As with any profession, some recruiters are more reputable than others. Therefore, as with any professional services, the best way to locate an appropriate recruiter for your job search is through a personal referral or recommendation. That means you should ask people who work in the same profession and specialty area that you are looking to work within. Let's say you wanted to work within the information technology industry as a nursing informatics specialist; ask anyone who works in the IT world who the good recruiters are in the industry, and they'll likely know or be able to find out. Likewise, if you wanted to work in the pharmaceutical industry, you could ask any pharmacist or drug salesperson. Chances are these people know because recruiters are in touch with them periodically.

Professional recruiters generally do not advertise their services to potential job candidates. That is because they do not necessarily want people who are looking for a job calling them. That does not mean you cannot make direct contact with a recruiter you wish to work with, but we'll discuss that more in a moment. Occasionally, a recruiter will place an ad for their services in the back of select professional journals and publications or select websites, usually those geared more toward managers and administrators. You can also look on the Internet using search terms, such as "health care search firms" or "executive search firms," to locate some.

Q: *Can I work with more than one recruiter?*

A: Yes, but not on the same job. It is possible that more than one search firm is working on the same professional opportunity. For example, you may already be interviewing, or being considered, for a position with a particular company through a search firm. You might be contacted by another search firm who discusses a certain position they are conducting a search for without mentioning the company or facility name. If the position sounds very similar to one you are already interviewing for, you should say something to the recruiter like, "Is this by any chance a position with County Medical?" The recruiter will either confirm that it is that position or advise you that it is not. If it is the same, you should advise this recruiter that you are already being considered for that position through another search firm.

A recruiter may ask you to enter into an exclusive arrangement with them—meaning you would not work with other search firms during a specified period of time. While you are under no obligation to do so, it can work to your advantage to agree to a short-term exclusivity contract of not more than 2 weeks. When you agree to this, the recruiter will often work extra hard during that time to find an appropriate position for you.

Q: *How do I approach a recruiter I'd like to work with?*

A: Once you've received a referral or recommendation for a particular recruiter or you've identified whom you want to contact, make an initial phone call or send an email. Introduce yourself, and explain what you're interested in. For example, you might say something like, "My name is Frank Miller. I'm a registered nurse interested in getting into health care sales and marketing. I think we might be able to help each other. Do you have a few moments to speak with me?" Be clear, concise, and direct in your communication. Be ready to sell yourself and tell the recruiter what distinguishes you from the crowd.

This would be the *wrong* way to approach a professional recruiter: "Hi, I'm an RN and I'm looking to do something different outside of the hospital." The recruiter would likely say, "Well, what are you looking to do?" And you answer, "I'm really not sure. I kinda want to see what's out there." That's a sure way to turn the recruiter off. In other words, you have to have some concept of what you're looking for or at least sound like you do.

If you're speaking to a recruiter who specializes in health care management positions and you're not sure what you're looking for, say something like, "I'm particularly interested in education positions but will consider any management level position." You must master assertive telephone skills. And since professional recruiters all have their own specialties, it is also helpful to add, after stating your interests and background, "Are you the right recruiter to speak with?" If they say they are not, ask them for a referral to another, better suited, recruiter.

If working with a professional recruiter does not sound like the right choice for your job search, you still have other options for getting some help, including using staffing and employment agencies.

Staffing and Employment Agencies

There are many types of agencies other than search firms that you might work with in seeking employment. Through these agencies, nurses can find per diem, part-time, temporary, contract, and even direct hire employment. Individuals who work in this industry may refer to themselves as recruiters, employment counselors, placement counselors, employment consultants, and staffing coordinators. Here are examples of different types of agencies.

Traditional nursing or health care staffing agencies. These agencies typically focus on nursing staffing in health care facilities and offer per diem and contract work. However, many staffing agencies also offer positions in alternate settings, such as school nursing, occupational health nursing, legal nurse consulting, nursing informatics, and others. Be sure to specifically ask about those other opportunities if you're interested in them.

Travel nurse agencies. Travel nurse agencies contract with nurses to take temporary assignments, on average 3 months at a time, in various parts of the country. Nurses can generally pick their own assignment regarding specialty and geographic location. Most travel nurse agencies will assist you in moving, finding housing, and getting a license to practice in your new location. I once met a nurse who worked for a travel nurse agency but only took assignments in her local area so she didn't have to travel at all. Of course, most nurses who work for travel nurse agencies do so because of the travel opportunity. Some agencies offer domestic as well as international assignments. For overseas assignments, the time commitment is longer, usually 6 months to 2 years in length.

Part-time and temporary health care agencies. Some health care employment agencies specialize exclusively in part-time and temporary, or "temp," work. Generally speaking, their focus is on positions away from the bedside, such as school nursing, occupational and public health nursing, opportunities in the pharmaceutical industry, and the like. A temp job could last for a few days to a year.

For those nurses specifically looking for part-time and occasional work in a nontraditional setting, this type of agency can be helpful. The advantage of working with a part-time or temp agency in particular is that it is a good opportunity to try out a nontraditional specialty to determine if you like it before making a full-time commitment. Also, it's a great way to gain some experience and get your foot in the door of a company or industry you'd like to transition into. Even if you are looking for full-time employment, many part-time and temp jobs turn into full-time or lead to other full-time positions within the company. So if, for example, you are considering working in occupational health or pharmaceutical research, but either can't get your foot in the door anywhere, or would like to try it before applying for a full-time job, part-time or temp employment through an agency is a good option.

General employment agencies. In addition to nursing and health care staffing agencies, there are some general employment agencies that

Helen is a recruiter with 20 years of experience in the employment industry, who works with both health care and non–health care job candidates. She offers the following advice to nurses:

"Appreciate the value you bring to the bigger health care industry. Some nurses come to me with no confidence in themselves. They undervalue their own skills and abilities and how those skills can be used in other industries and other settings beyond the hospital.

"If you get blown off by a company you wish to work for, ask if they use temps or consultants. If they say they do, ask, 'Which agency do you work with?' Temping is a great way to get a foot in the door and gain valuable experience.

"When working with an agency, be flexible with your expectations and be open-minded about opportunities and salaries. Some candidates are very rigid and say, 'This is who I am, and this is what I want.' You may be cutting yourself off from some great opportunities."

occasionally have positions for health care professionals, both regular and temporary. Be sure to explore all sources.

The best way to find an agency of any type is through referral or word of mouth. Ask around and see who has worked with which agencies. Of course, most nursing agencies advertise in nursing publications, both print and online. And don't forget that agencies of all types exhibit at career and job fairs and conventions. It's a great chance to get up close and personal with recruiters.

Almost all nurse staffing agencies, including travel nurse agencies, require that a nurse have at least 1–2 years of general patient care experience. That is because an agency nurse needs to hit the ground running in any assignment, adapt quickly to a new environment, and be able to work very independently. There is no orientation or preceptor and sometimes limited access to support systems. While newly licensed nurses might be able to find nontraditional nursing work through an agency, they would not be considered qualified for a traditional patient care assignment here.

Many health care facilities and companies have their own in-house recruiters who recruit for all levels of positions within the company while others recruit for specific types of positions only. This includes hospitals, pharmaceutical companies, and others. If there are particular facilities or companies you wish to work for, try making direct contact with that recruiter via telephone or email and via LI.

While recruiters work on connecting prospective employees with employers, some firms can facilitate the job search process in other ways.

Career Management and Outplacement Firms

We discussed career management services in chapter 3 in relation to helping you decide what you want to do. Outplacement firms, career coaches, and counselors do not place you in positions but can assist you in the job search process. They may even have important contacts to help you along. Just be sure to understand the difference between a professional recruiter or agency who will directly hook you up with employers at no cost to you and a career management firm that will primarily assist you with self-marketing and career focus for a fee, though sometimes that fee is paid by your employer as the result of a layoff or facility closing.

Using Volunteering as a Job Search Tool

By now you've noticed that various career management tools and techniques have more than one purpose. The same holds true for volunteering. Not only can volunteering provide some great experience, it can also be an effective job-finding tool. If there is a specialty or an employer you really want to work for but haven't had any luck with through traditional channels, consider offering to volunteer there. Volunteering not only provides an opportunity to gain relevant experience, but it often leads to paid employment. Here are some real-life examples of how other nurses used volunteering, some unwittingly, to land the job of their dreams.

Karen was a staff nurse for 15 years. She had done some career research and decided that she wanted to break into QI. She applied for a few job openings she saw advertised online but wasn't getting any calls. She decided to approach the director of the QI department in her current place of employment. She inquired about openings but was told none existed at present. So she offered to volunteer 2 hours per week for them. She agreed to do whatever was necessary, even filing and answering the phone. She was desperate to get any exposure she could to the specialty. Lo and behold, 4 months down the road, a full-time position became available for a QI nurse. The job wasn't even advertised yet and was offered to Karen. Why? Because she was already there, they knew her, and the transition was a breeze. Karen happily accepted the position. Although she never expected a job offer when initially offering to volunteer, her initiative paid big dividends.

Alyce was a very accomplished nurse working in a very narrow and highly specialized field. She had worked in her specialty for many years, held leadership positions in her national professional association, and was once editor of a journal in her specialty. She had worked her way to the top of her field and was quite content. One day she was notified that her department was being eliminated and she was being laid off. "I never saw it coming," she said. "It felt like the rug had been pulled out from under me. I panicked, wondering where I could possibly go from here. There were so few good positions available in my specialty, and the thought of starting over again at my age [58 years] was unfathomable." Alyce had been unemployed for almost a year when she attended one of my Career Alternatives for Nurses seminars. Three months after the seminar, Alyce contacted me with some exciting news. "I would have never thought of using volunteering as a job search technique before coming to your seminar. And honestly, I didn't really believe it would work. But I took your advice and thought about my ideal work situation. There was a facility I had always dreamed of working for, so I decided to contact them inquiring about a position in my specialty. They didn't have any openings when I called, so I told them I'd like to volunteer there anyway. Here I was sitting at home doing nothing and not getting paid. I figured I might as well do something constructive, even if not getting paid. They were rather startled by my offer and said no one had ever offered to volunteer there before." Alyce became a volunteer for 4 hours a week at her dream employer. Three months later, a part-time position opened up, and it was automatically offered to Alyce. She was told that the job would likely turn into a full-time position by the end of the year. Needless to say, she was ecstatic.

Carrie was a registered nurse and certified personal trainer. When she contacted me, she had been working exclusively as a personal trainer for several years and wanted to also utilize her nursing background. I suggested she look into cardiac rehabilitation, which combines nursing and fitness. She was very interested in the prospect but didn't feel she could just jump back into the clinical arena after an absence of several years. So I suggested she volunteer at a cardiac rehab center for a while to get her bearings as this is a low-risk way to reenter health care. After a few months as a volunteer there, she was feeling comfortable and confident and applied for a position in the department. They were thrilled to have her, and she found a way to combine her two loves: fitness and nursing.

Some Additional Job-Finding Tips

When actively seeking employment, it is necessary for prospective employers to be able to contact you easily. Be sure to have an email address that is neutral and professional, such as fmccarthy@nnn.net. Examples of unprofessional email addresses are hotchicknurse@nnn.net and pooh-bearkisses@nnn.net. Check your email and phone messages often and be sure that neither gets full or starts rejecting incoming messages. If you have a spam filter on your email account, be sure to scan rejected emails to be certain a legitimate message didn't get inadvertently bumped into that folder, which happens all the time.

If no one is available to accept a phone call and the caller can't leave a message, it can make prospective employers or recruiters crazy if they're trying to reach you to set up an interview. If they call you even once, get no answer, and have no capacity to leave a message, they may not call again.

Be sure to have a professional message on your voice mail, too, at least while you're in the job market. Playing music or reciting a poem, having your children speak the message in unison, or saying something glib can be a turnoff to someone who doesn't know you yet.

Sample Letter of Introduction for Informational Interviewing

©Donna Cardillo. Reprinted with permission.

Carl Frazier, RN, BSN
200 Main Street
Crystal Cave, NJ 88094
732-555-0986
cfrazier@nnn.net

May 7, 20 __

Janet Fredericks, RN, MSN
Chief Nursing Officer
State of New Jersey Department of Health Affairs
22 Main Street
Trenton, NJ 88007

Dear Ms. Fredericks,

Carol Edwards of County General Hospital suggested I contact you. She said you were top in your field and would be a great person for me to speak with. Congratulations on your career success! Like you, I am a registered nurse with a pediatric background. I am exploring my career options and am interested in working for state government.

I would appreciate the opportunity to meet briefly with you in person, at your convenience, and learn more about you and how you got started in your current career path. I'm also interested in learning more about what other nurses are doing in the Department of Health Affairs.

I will contact you in the next week in the hopes that we can set up an appointment. In the meantime, if you care to reach me, my cell phone is 732-555-8994.

Sincerely,

Carl Frazier, RN, BSN

Carl Frazier, RN, BSN

Sample Marketing Letter
Sample Letter One
©Donna Cardillo. Reprinted with permission.

Carl Frazier, RN, BSN
200 Main Street
Crystal Cave, NJ 88094
732-555-0986
cfrazier@nnn.net

November 8, 20 __

Frederick Castle
Director, Health Services
College Health Plan
44 Alleghany Road
West Crawford, TX 88094

Dear Mr. Castle,

I'm seeking an administrative level position with College Health Plan. As a health care professional, I appreciate the role that managed care plays in keeping their members healthy and well. Always looking to stay ahead of the curve, I realize that a large managed care company offers exactly the type of opportunities I am looking for. College Health Plan is a leader in the managed care industry, and I've got my sights set on being a part of that winning team.

I am a registered nurse with more than 20 years of progressive clinical and managerial experience. I have been involved in project management, human resource management, new program development, and services marketing. In addition to solid and diverse experience, I possess great problem-solving and conflict management skills. I also have an innate ability to motivate and energize those around me, and I am passionate about health care in general. I would be an asset to your company.

Not only would I relish the opportunity to work under an established industry leader like yourself, but I would be privileged to become a part of your dynamic and growing company. I will contact you within the next week so that we can discuss our mutual interests further.

Very Truly Yours,

Carl Frazier, RN, BSN

Carl Frazier, RN, BSN

Sample Marketing Letter
Sample Letter Two
©Donna Cardillo. Reprinted with permission.

Janice Smith, RN, MSN
45 Lane Avenue
Smithville, NJ 00090
732-555-0220
jsmith@nnn.net

October 30, 20__

Mary Harris, RN, MSN
Director of Quality Management
Allenwood Medical Center
311 City Street
Allenwood, NJ 22536

Dear Ms. Harris,

I am interested in working for Allenwood Medical Center as a Quality Improvement Coordinator. I am attracted by Allenwood's reputation for quality and service, and I am confident I can contribute to that.

As an RN with more than 15 years of critical care experience, I possess excellent clinical, managerial, and technical skills. I have also developed good communication skills while interacting with physicians, patients, and other health care professionals in a variety of situations. As a result of my committee work and my involvement in nursing quality improvement, I have developed a keen interest in hospital-wide quality management activities and have decided to pursue this career path.

In summary, I can offer you solid clinical experience, the ability to work well with all types of people, as well as energy and enthusiasm. I am willing to start in an entry-level position and learn from the bottom up. I am a quick study and determined to become an outcomes management professional.

I look forward to meeting with you so that we can discuss our mutual interests further. I will call you in one week to follow up.

Sincerely,

Janice Smith, RN, MSN

Janice Smith, RN, MSN

Chapter 5

Your Résumé

A résumé is a key self-marketing tool, yet very few nurses have an effective one. Why? Many of us have never taken the time to learn the correct way to develop one. Also, many of us are intimidated by the process and are uncomfortable writing about ourselves in a positive way. Many nurses, especially those who have been in the same job for an extended period of time, have never had any type of résumé. There was a time when nurses didn't even need one; our license to practice was all that was required to be hired. But, of course, those days are long gone and every nurse needs a professional résumé ready to go at a moment's notice.

Note: A résumé and curriculum vitae (CV) are two entirely different documents used in different settings. I'll discuss CVs in chapter 6.

The purpose of a résumé is to highlight your more interesting, significant, and marketable skills and experiences. It is a synopsis of your credentials, achievements, skill set, and work history. It is a snapshot of your entire career. Therefore, the goal of effective résumé writing is to maximize your experience on paper and put your best foot forward. You do not need to enumerate everything you ever did or reveal everything there is to know about you. Rather, you want to develop a document that conveys the best of your background and presents it in the best possible light. You want to pique the reader's interest. Think of it as an advertisement or brochure for a product or service, where the selling points are highlighted, not all of the specifics given.

Résumés are not used just for changing jobs. They may be requested when applying for a promotion or transfer, putting in a proposal to speak or present a poster at a conference, applying for a position on the board of a professional association, submitting an article for publication, or various other reasons. And, as previously discussed, you may be very happily employed now, but you never know when your employment situation will change, your needs will change, or an opportunity will present itself that you had not previously considered. For example, you might have an opportunity to do some part-time consulting while you maintain your current position and a prospective client or employer might want to see your résumé or keep a copy on file. The point is if someone asks you for your résumé, you want to have one ready, not be scrambling to develop one at the last minute only to find that your printer is out of ink. Besides, it makes sense to keep an up-to-date, written record of your work experience and accomplishments. It is so easy to forget what you've done otherwise, especially as the years pass. Imagine suddenly needing a résumé when you don't have a current one and having to recall and construct, on short notice, 10 years' worth of accomplishments and experiences. It has happened to many of us and it is not a pretty sight! Nor is the resulting résumé.

Even in this digital age of online applications, hard copy résumés still have a place and are great marketing tools in many situations. But whether posting online or presenting a hard copy, your résumé still needs to meet contemporary standards and stand out from the crowd in a good way.

By now it should be clear that if you don't have a résumé, it is time to develop one. If you do have one, chances are it needs to be updated and reformatted to reflect current résumé writing standards and to best show-case your unique background. And while most people break into a cold sweat at the thought of having to develop a résumé, the process is actually much less difficult once you understand the purpose and learn the correct format and style of résumé writing. Let's review the basics. Examples are given at the end of the chapter.

Format
There are essentially three different types of résumés: chronological, functional, and combination. All three have a unique purpose and differ in the way that information is presented. Let's take a closer look at each.

Chronological

The chronological résumé (example 1) is the most commonly used and the one most people are familiar with. It focuses on work experience and starts with the current or most recent position and works its way back from there. It lists each job with several bullet points of related information. This is the type that is preferred by most recruiters and prospective employers. It tells a story and shows progression of employment history.

Functional

A functional résumé (example 2) shifts the focus to categories of experience and downplays individual jobs and work history. For example, a functional résumé would group experience by categories such as teaching, writing, researching, sales and marketing, and clinical. It might also include a general category, "Selected Accomplishments," for those things that the writer wishes to highlight beyond the experience categories. This type of résumé is best used by either someone with extensive, exceptional, or unique experience who has been out of the workforce for a while or someone who is looking to totally change gears in their career, such as going from clinical work to education. A consultant who is working independently might also use it. A prospective client is more interested in a consultant's relevant work experience than in their work history. A functional résumé might also be an option for someone with a very erratic work history who may need or want to shift the focus away from an employment record to their strengths and abilities.

I once coached a nurse who had been out of the workforce for 10 years while raising a family. Before that, she had exceptional work experience in management and education. She also had outstanding credentials and many impressive accomplishments. She was an ideal candidate for a functional résumé.

We worked together to compose a dynamite document that highlighted her strengths while downplaying her absence from the workforce. This type of résumé not only made the nurse feel more confident, but it was effective in getting her several interviews and ultimately an excellent position as the director of educational services for a social service agency.

I do not mean to imply that the functional format should automatically be used in the above-mentioned examples or that everyone who has been out of the workforce for a while should use it. That simply is not the case. The point is that the functional format may be a useful alternative to the chronological format in certain situations.

The theory behind the functional format is that it forces the reader (recruiter, client, or prospective employer) to focus on experience rather than dates and length of employment. If you can impress the reader on page one with your experiences and accomplishments, by the time they get to the second page, your work history is deemphasized. Of course this theory is debatable.

On the downside, because some people use the functional résumé to downplay a problematic work history, the functional format makes some prospective employers suspicious. And because many employers are simply accustomed to the chronological format and prefer it, they get annoyed with this format. The bottom line is, consider your own unique background and career goals, and choose the format that best serves your needs.

Combination

This is a combination of formats (résumé sample 3 at end of chapter) that might be used by a consultant, someone in a very specialized field, or someone with unique and extensive experience. It generally combines elements of the chronological and functional résumés as well as the CV and would be typically longer than the average résumé, which is one to two pages. A combination résumé could feasibly be three to four pages in length.

When I went into business as a speaker, writer, and consultant, I shifted to a combination style of résumé, a cross between a functional résumé and a CV. Neither format was exactly right for me, so I took elements of both to create a document that worked for me. My clients are interested in specific types of experiences I have (speaking, writing, teaching) rather than my employment history. However, a simple functional résumé would not do in my case because I also have numerous publications, speaking credentials, awards, and professional association involvement. I use a four-page combination format to best showcase my background and credentials.

Note: When submitting a résumé online you may not have these choices. Follow the instructions on the individual web site where you are submitting. That being said, you should always have hard copy résumés available to bring to interviews, career fairs, and professional networking events. Hard copies can also be sent via post mail as a follow-up to online submissions.

Layout and Writing Style

Today's prospective employers visually scan, rather than read, résumés. This means they give it an initial quick look-over to see if some basic elements are there or if anything catches their attention. It is said that the average résumé reader scans a résumé in 3–20 seconds. What can they glean in that short amount of time? If written and organized well, they should be able to tell if you have the basic experience and credentials they are looking for. At the very least, they should be intrigued enough to want to read or scan more.

With that in mind, you should create a résumé in a high-impact style; that is, one that is well organized, concise, upbeat, and laid out to make information easy to find and scan and hopefully read. The layout of your résumé should be consistent throughout the document.

The following are important characteristics of a high-impact style of writing.

Use a Bulleted Format

Each piece of information or sound bite in the "Experience" section of a chronological résumé or "Selected Accomplishments" section of a functional résumé should be preceded by a large dot or bullet in a list format. This style makes it easy for the eyes to scan, and it effectively showcases what you want the reader to focus on. Be sure to use a bullet point instead of a diamond, arrow, star, asterisk, or other distracting symbol. List one accomplishment or responsibility per bullet. The narrative for each bullet should ideally be on one to two lines maximum. If it gets longer than that, it becomes laborious to read. Edit to reduce the phrases and sentence(s) as needed.

Make It Lively

Start each bullet point with an action verb for an upbeat, active tone (see "Action Verbs for Your Résumé" on pages 124–125). In other words, rather than preceding each statement with "responsible for" or "involved in," use more proactive language such as "initiated," "directed," and "oversaw." Example: The item, "Responsible for orientation of new hires," reads better as, "Oriented and trained new hires." You're not claiming to be the only one who does this; you're simply describing your activities in a more assertive, action-oriented way.

Brevity Is Key

Use short, truncated sentences rather than complete sentences. By eliminating unnecessary words and phrases, you assist the reader in focusing in on what is important and significant. Examples follow below:

- **Too wordy:** Administered primary nurse case management in home care setting to adults by assessing, developing, implementing, and evaluating each patient's plan of care.
- **More concise:** Conducted adult case management in home care setting.
- **Too wordy:** Coordinated all aspects of clinical drug study, including data collection, accurate maintenance of records according to study protocol, completion of case report forms, and interaction with physicians.
- **More concise:** Coordinated all aspects of clinical drug studies.

Use Clear Headings

Create category headings ("EXPERIENCE," "EDUCATION," etc.) in uppercase letters and bold print so they are easy to spot. Position all headings in the same place throughout the document, either in the center of the page or to the far left (flush left). This way the readers can quickly find what they're looking for.

Be Clear and Specific

Keep the language simple and clear throughout. Avoid vague and generalized statements such as "Initiated plan of care with recommendations to physicians and provided ongoing progress assessments," or "Another facet of my position is to interface with physicians and all staff members to allow the patient a positive perioperative experience." Not only are both of these statements vague, they relate to very basic, routine duties, which do not belong on your résumé.

Here's an example of a confusing statement: "Utilized dynamic, interpersonal, and negotiation talents to develop and maintain cohesive relationships with hospital discharge planners, thereby substantially expanding and diversifying the source of temporary employment vacancies from supplemental positions within hospitals to home care opportunities." Interestingly enough, this statement appeared on a functional résumé under the heading of "Communication Skills." Not only is the sentence wordy and complex, but the reader would be hard-pressed to understand its meaning. I was exhausted just reading it.

Résumé Content

Later in this chapter ("How to Develop and Update Your Résumé"), we'll discuss how to gather the information needed to start developing your résumé content. Right now, we'll discuss how to choose that which is most important and interesting in your background and how to present it in the best possible light. Here are some general guidelines for developing content.

Be Selective

When choosing what to include on your résumé, less is more. Everyone is on information overload these days so you don't need to mention everything you've ever done. When describing work experiences, avoid routine duties and focus on that which is most important and interesting.

Expand Your Vision

Show a diversity of experience (see skills and experience inventory sidebar at the end of the chapter); don't focus on clinical skills alone as that is only one aspect of what a nurse does. Include any speaking or writing you did, business or managerial experience acquired, special projects worked on, interprofessional committees you sat on, and so on. If you are a new nurse or worked off-shifts or per diem and therefore have had limited experiences beyond the clinical, at least enhance or "punch up" the description of your clinical skills. For example, "IV certified, proficient in ventilator management, conducted patient and family teaching," sounds much better than: "Picked up doctor's orders, delivered patient meds, took vital signs." Your résumé should not read like a job description.

Spell It Out

Don't use undefined acronyms, making your résumé an alphabet soup. Remember, many people in other specialties may not know the acronyms common in your specialty. Even if you are applying for a job in the same specialty you currently work in, human resource (HR) professionals will likely be reading and screening your résumé before it gets to someone in your specialty. If the HR people can't understand it, they may disregard it. The general rule when using an acronym is to spell it out the first time you use it. Example: "cardiac step-down unit (CSDU)." After that, you can use the acronym throughout the document.

Show Progression of Responsibility
Demonstrate an increase in responsibility and position when possible. For example, if you were originally hired as a staff nurse and later promoted to charge nurse, rather than listing both positions separately list it once as:

- Hired as staff nurse. After two years, promoted to shift supervisor. One year later, promoted to nurse manager.

Then, proceed to list bullet points of information related to your highest level of authority. Of course, you can include significant experiences or accomplishments from your original positions too, as long as you don't overdo it.

Focus on the Here and Now
The older the position is, the less you need to say about it. Your résumé should focus on the most recent and most important information. (See "Frequently Asked Questions" section of this chapter about how far back to go on your résumé.)

Pump It Up with Numbers
Use quantitative data (numbers or percentages) whenever possible to demonstrate scope of responsibility, especially in supervisory and administrative roles, such as:

- Dollar amount of the budget you managed,
- Number and type of staff you were responsible for,
- Size of unit or facility worked in (number of beds, volume of outpatient visits per year), and
- What your sales volume was.

Show Results
Use quantitative data as applicable to demonstrate results achieved, such as:

- Percentage decrease of undesirable outcomes, such as infections, falls, or staff turnover attributable to special projects and policies you developed or implemented; and

- Percentage increase of desirable results, such as increased sales volume.

Don't Repeat Yourself

If you did essentially the same thing at more than one place of employment, don't list identical bullet points of information under both jobs. That is boring and redundant. Try to vary the wording and the description if possible.

Key Elements

Organize your résumé in a way that makes it easy for the reader to quickly find whatever information they are looking for. It should be broken down into general categories and should contain certain basic information. Following is information about how to maximize each section of your résumé so the information works to your best advantage.

Identifying Information

At the top of the first page of your résumé, include your name, credentials, address, cell phone number, and email address. You can also include your home phone number although many just use a cell these days. It's ideal to list only the number that makes you most accessible. Consider including your LinkedIn URL as well, but only if your profile is up to date. At the top of subsequent pages, it is only necessary to include your name and page number. Suggestion: Put your name in bold print to make it stand out.

Objective versus Summary

Contrary to what you may have heard, it is not necessary to include an objective on your résumé. They are even considered passé by some. Additionally, an objective can actually work against you. Here's why.

Most people use one of two types of objectives. The first is position-specific, such as "Looking for a position in case management." The problem with this is that if you apply for another type of position, you will have to redo your résumé to amend or remove that statement. This is not practical or always even possible because of time constraints. Besides, if you're applying for a case management job, it should be fairly obvious that your objective is to find a position in case management. And, since a cover letter would normally accompany a résumé that is mailed, faxed, or emailed (unless you are specifically advised *not* to send a cover letter), that would be the place to mention which specific position you are applying for or what your areas of interest are.

The other type of objective consists of a flowery statement that says something general like: "Looking for a position where I can utilize all of my skills and abilities to deliver excellent patient care." This statement is vague, general, and virtually meaningless. So what's the point?

Remember that you have only 3–20 seconds to grab the interest and attention of the reader. And since the first few lines on your résumé are the first thing the reader is likely to look at, you want it to be strong, energizing, and interesting.

Note: If attending a career fair or facility open house where a cover letter is not customarily used, you can mention to the recruiter if you have a particular preference for position or department.

A good alternative to the objective is the summary. I am not referring to a summary of qualifications that some people use where they list, in summary form, what's already in their résumé. Rather, I am referring to a short paragraph made up of two to three powerful, punchy sentences or phrases that represent the best you have to offer. The first sentence should give an overview of your experience. The second and third sentences should convey strong personality traits, one or two exceptional skills or abilities, and other desirable attributes.

Here are a few examples:

- RN with unique background combining both health care and business experience. Excellent teaching and training skills. Detail-oriented, energetic, and creative problem solver. Social media and technology savvy.

- Newly licensed nurse brimming with enthusiasm and drive. Possesses a good work ethic and a strong desire to be a successful professional nurse. Has developed excellent communication skills and is not afraid to ask questions or ask for help as needed.

- LPN with more than 25 years of diverse experience in acute care, long-term care, and community health. Conscientious clinician who loves direct patient care as much as supervision and training. Considered a team player and self-starter.

- Seasoned administrator with a proven record of streamlining inefficient operations and creating profitable departments. Well versed in regulatory affairs. Considered approachable, fair-minded, and results-oriented.

- Experienced nurse educator who is passionate about teaching. Accomplished writer, speaker, and trainer. Creative, high-energy, and very organized professional with a great sense of humor.

This type of summary serves as an introduction to you. The examples above are high-energy and grab the reader's attention. They draw the reader in, provide a good feeling about the candidate, and make them want to read more and hopefully learn more about you by bringing you in for an interview. And while some may criticize the use of clichés such as "team-player" and "self-starter," the truth is that these phrases are still commonly used by employers and recruiters in classified ads, job descriptions, and interviews and elicit a positive response from potential employers.

Employer Information

List the employer's name followed by city and state. It is not necessary to include a complete address for each employer on your résumé. If a prospective employer wants that information, they'll ask you to provide it on an application or reference form. It is a good idea to put the employer's name in bold print so that it stands out.

Your Title

List your current or last title held under the employer's name followed by the department(s) or unit(s) if applicable. Consider putting your title in italics to make it stand out from the rest of the print. If you were a staff nurse or unit manager on more than one unit but with similar responsibilities, you can list the title once, followed by the units. For example: *Staff Nurse, Orthopedics, Medical-Surgical, Telemetry*.

If you've had several different titles, positions, or both over the years with the same employer, list the titles separately unless they describe promotions within the same department. In this case, list the employer's name only once with total years of employment there. When listing each position, put the years associated with it in parentheses right next to the title. For example:

Country Side Medical Center, Calico, NY   2010–2016
Unit Manager, Psychiatry (2010–2014)

Include a position overview (see below) and several bullet points as appropriate. Repeat this method with subsequent titles at the same place of employment.

Position Overview

If using a chronological résumé, under each position listed in the experience section, give a one-sentence overview that conveys the scope of responsibility or a general description of the type of work you did (see résumé sample 1 at end of chapter).

Employment Dates

List dates of employment either to the right of the employer's name or to the left; either way is technically correct, however listing them to the right of the page is preferable for several reasons. Since we read from left to right, our eyes automatically scan the left side of the page first. Therefore, listing dates of employment on the right forces the reader to focus on your experience and accomplishments rather than your dates of employment.

It is not necessary to use an exact dates of employment start and stop, but only the year. For example, if you worked somewhere from January 3, 2014, to August 4, 2016, you only need to state "2014–2016." If you worked from January to December of 2013, just put "2013." This can help to smooth out some rough edges on your résumé if you have trouble spots with your dates. Besides, employers don't want or need that much information on your résumé.

Note: Don't confuse filling out a job application with developing a professional résumé. They are two entirely different documents. If an employer asks you to fill out an application, which requires the month of employment start and stop, then you can provide that information on the application. However, since every employer is different, when asked to fill out a job application, ask, "Can I just attach my résumé?" If they ask you to also fill out the application, ask if you need to complete the whole thing or just certain parts. Since both documents are used in different ways, comply with whatever they request.

Note: Once you become self-employed or if you are working as a consultant, you can eliminate the dates of employment on a functional résumé.

Categories

In addition to work experience, traditional résumé categories include education, licenses and certifications, special skills, professional affiliations, and community and volunteer work, not necessarily in that order. Additional categories, such as awards and honors, publications, presentations, and military service, may be used if applicable. Following are some guidelines for each.

Licenses and Certifications

List all professional licenses you carry in any state. For example, if you are applying for a job in Maryland and hold Maryland and California nursing licenses, list them both. It is not necessary to list your actual nursing license number or years of issue and expiration on your résumé.

Only list current information; no one is interested in what certifications or licenses you've had in the past if they have lapsed for reasons other than disciplinary actions. It is also not necessary to list the date you first became certified in something. Too many irrelevant details clog up your résumé.

Remember to spell out certification acronyms. For example, certified emergency nurse (CEN). If you only list the acronym and the reader doesn't know what it stands for, then you might as well leave it off your résumé for all the good it will do. You may want to include the organization that issued the certification, but this is optional.

Education

List your highest level of education first and work your way down from there. If you are currently enrolled in school for a higher degree, put that first to highlight that you are pursuing a higher degree as follows:

City College
Master's degree in nursing—currently pursuing

Be sure to include all of your degrees, including nonnursing degrees.

If you took a certain number of credits at a college, but never finished the degree and are not currently active in the program, you can state it this way:

City College—32 graduate level credits completed

Of course, it is advisable to enroll in even one course so that you can say "currently pursuing" as above and indicate you are working toward completion.

If you started your degree program in one school and finished it up in another, it is only necessary to list the school that issued your diploma.

There is no need to note the start date of any educational experience. There is also no need to include the date you graduated from any educational program unless you are a newly licensed nurse. Likewise, it is not necessary to include anticipated graduation dates for education unless you are a student nurse in a basic nursing education program. This does not apply to licensed nurses who are advancing their education (see "Special Situations" later in the chapter).

If you received school-related honors or special recognition such as cum laude or other academic awards, you should include them. However, it is not necessary to include a list of academic scholarships.

High school information generally is not included on a professional résumé, with a few exceptions. If you had outstanding or unusual achievements demonstrating leadership, community service, or notable academic accomplishments, you might consider adding them. I once coached a nurse who had a swimming scholarship named after her in high school because of her leadership abilities. That is an honor worth noting and makes a very positive statement about the nurse. Therefore, we decided to include this information on her résumé under "Awards and Honors."

If you are a newly licensed nurse and attended nursing school right out of high school, it could be beneficial to initially include select information from high school years on your résumé, such as being a member or officer of a Future Nurses of America Club, or if you were a member of a health care association, such as Health Occupations Students of America (HOSA).

However, once you cease to be a new nurse (1–2 years after graduation, regardless of experience), this type of information is no longer relevant and should be removed from your résumé.

It is not advisable to list continuing education (CE) credits here. That's because a laundry list of CE courses taken only serves to clutter up your résumé. Employers are primarily concerned with your formal education and degrees. You can mention any relevant CE courses in your cover letter or on an interview. If you really want to, you can write something here, such as, "Continuing education courses [or credits] available upon request," to indicate that you have taken them. However, this is not necessary.

Special Skills

This is the place to highlight special skills and abilities, beyond that which is already on your résumé, such as basic and advanced social media, computer, or other technology skills, languages spoken and written, good writing and speaking skills, and so on.

Awards and Honors

List special recognition you have received from employers, professional associations, or your community, including attendance awards, nurse of the year, service awards, and so on. As an alternative, employment-related awards can be listed as a bullet point under a specific job in work history.

Professional Affiliations

List professional associations you currently belong to. Spell out the name of the organizations listed. There is no need to include the date you joined the organization. It is not necessary to list offices held in the past unless you are a past president. Be selective about including current leadership positions held as well as special projects and committees worked on. If you have other professional association experience, past or present, that is relevant to a job you are applying for, you can mention that in your cover letter. For example, if you are applying for a job in education, you can mention in your cover letter that you were active on the education committee of an association and elaborate on the types of things you did that are relevant to this position. However, you can also reserve that for mention on the interview. It can be nice to have something a little extra to offer to add value.

When listing an organization whose name is not self-explanatory, such as Sigma (previously Sigma Theta Tau International [STTI]), it is advisable to add an explanatory phrase such as "honor society for nursing," since many people, including other nurses, do not know what that is. Remember, if the reader doesn't know what something is or what it means, the information is meaningless.

Publications

If you have published work, by all means list that. This would include articles published online or in print publications, chapters written for books, and so forth. If you have only one or two published works, list them under the heading "Publications." If you have more than a few, it's best to use the heading "Selected Publications." This indicates that what you have listed is a sampling of what you've written but that there is more. List only a few of the most recent or more significant works under this heading. A full listing, along with a writing sample, can always be submitted separately if requested. It is not necessary to list these publications in full bibliography format on a résumé (see résumé example 2 at end of chapter).

Presentations

If you have done a few major presentations at conferences, conventions, and career fairs, list them under the heading "Presentations." As with publications, use "Selected Presentations" if the list is longer. Presentations might be listed in this way:

> "Managing the Patient with Type I Diabetes." Arkansas Nurses Association Annual Convention 2016.

Presentations done as part of one's employment can be included in summary form as a bullet point under that place of employment. For example:

- Presents regularly at in-service sessions, new employee orientation, and community outreach programs on topics such as management of diabetes, foot care, and nutrition.

Volunteer and Community Work

Be selective but do include those activities, both past and present, that demonstrate leadership and other important skills and experiences as well as civic involvement. Be sure to include all health care–related volunteer experience and work with youth groups, the elderly, the homeless, and so on. However, be cautious in listing work with organizations that would reveal your religious or political affiliations such as the Young Democrats of America or Right-to-Life Group. Aside from being personal and possibly prohibited from being asked under state or federal laws against discrimination, this type of information can work against you.

Military Service

List the type of duty you did (active or reserves), the branch of the service, your rank, and the type of work you did. Include any special commendations or medals.

What Not to Put on Your Résumé

When it comes to your résumé, some things are best left unsaid. Unnecessary and inappropriate information can make you look unsophisticated and unprofessional. It can also serve to distract the reader from your accomplishments and more important information. Here are several examples of things best left off your résumé.

Don't list hobbies like sewing, reading, or skiing. While a few prospective employers may claim this gives them insight into your personality, most recruiters find it too folksy and even irksome. The exception is for activities that reflect positively on you, such as having formerly competed in a particular sport, such as running a marathon or winning related awards, even on a local level. These might be mentioned in you cover letter or listed on your résumé under "Additional Information" or "Other Accomplishments."

Don't list personal information such as health status, height, and weight. This has no place on your professional résumé.

Don't list your age or marital status. This is protected information under current employment laws.

Don't list where or when you went to high school. It is considered irrelevant. However, there are exceptions, as there are to every rule. If, for example, you are a fairly new nurse and you attended a vocational or technical high school where you were trained as a nurse's aide or other caregiver, then it would be appropriate to list that education (see "Education" section above) at least until you've accumulated significant graduate nurse experience.

Don't list any salary information on your résumé. We'll get into when and how to discuss salary in chapters 7 and 8, but suffice to say it doesn't belong on your résumé.

Don't write "References available upon request" at the bottom of your résumé or list actual references with contact information in the body of your résumé. It is understood that if an employer wants references, they will ask for them, and you will supply them. If you don't, you don't get the job. End of story.

Don't type the word "résumé" on the top of the document (I've seen this more times than I can count). If the prospective employer can't figure out that it's a résumé by looking at it, then you have more serious problems.

The point is that you want to eliminate everything that is unnecessary from your résumé, decluttering it.

Appearance

First impressions are important in your personal appearance and so too in your résumé. That is why your résumé must be picture perfect. Its overall look will make an impression before the reader even reads one word. Here's what you need to know.

Paper

Use good quality 8 1/2 × 11 bond paper. Bond paper has high cotton fiber content and is used for stationary, as opposed to copy machine or computer paper. Choose a paper that looks and feels good. It should be 20 lb weight (which denotes the thickness and body of the paper, using bulk measurements) and have a watermark (an embedded logo visible when held up the light). Either linen or a flat finish (surface) is appropriate. Ask your local printer to show you some samples of good quality résumé paper. Be cautious of boxed paper labeled "résumé paper" in some office supply chains; often this is lower-grade, coarse paper and not professional in look or feel.

Color

Stick to white or off-white paper. Although gray or cream color is generally considered acceptable, it can appear muddy when the document is photocopied or electronically scanned.

Print

Only use black ink. Black print on white paper creates the best contrast for easy readability and makes a very professional-looking document. The print quality must be crisp, dark, and clear. Therefore, every copy of your résumé should be individually printed on a letter-quality laser printer, not photocopied. If you do not have such a printer, have your résumé printed by someone who does or bring it on a thumb drive to your local print shop or stationary store for printing. If the print on your résumé is fuzzy, light, or of otherwise poor quality, it will be difficult to read and may be disregarded and discarded. Print on only one side of the paper.

Character Size and Style

The type size (size of the letters) should be 12 point. Anything smaller is difficult to read. If the recruiter can't read it, it may wind up in the trash. And since many employers electronically scan résumés for paperless storage, 12-point type is preferable for scanning. Stick with an easily readable font such as Times New Roman.

Length

Résumés should be one to two pages in length on average. There is a common myth that nursing résumés should be on one page, but that has never been the case. By the time you list even one job along with your education and credentials, you're already on two pages, which is perfectly acceptable. On rare occasions, I would recommend a three-page résumé for someone with exceptional and extensive experience and credentials, but that would be the exception rather than the rule. Remember, less is more when it comes to résumé writing.

Margins

Margins should be approximately one inch on the top, bottom, and sides of each page of your résumé. You can alter those dimensions slightly, if necessary, but don't get carried away. If you need a bit more space on the page, it is better to reduce the top and bottom margins than the side margins. The empty space beyond the margins and anywhere that there is no printing is known as "white space." White space makes the printed part of the sheet easier to read and comprehend.

I once saw a résumé where the print literally took up the entire surface on the page. There were no margins at all. This nurse had heard that your résumé should be on one page, so he figured if he eliminated the margins, he could cram more information on one page. This is simply not acceptable. Not only is a document without margins difficult to follow, but it is completely unprofessional.

Some additional tips: Keep all information about one employer on the same page if possible. In other words, if you list a particular employer toward the bottom of the first page, try to list all information related to that employment on that page rather than continuing it on the second page. The exception would be if you held multiple positions or titles in that place of employment and simply can't fit it all on the first page. In that case, you could list the employer's name again at the top of the second page followed by "(continued)" and start with a new position held at that place of employment. In other words, don't split information about one employer, or at least not about one job title, onto two pages, if you can help it.

Stay away from fancy borders, designs, clip art, or background images on your résumé, such as shooting stars, flowers, clouds, or a caduceus (I've seen all of these). There is no place for this on a professional résumé, and it only serves to distract the reader.

Do not staple, tape, or paperclip the pages of your résumé together.

Special Situations

There are some situations that require special handling on your résumé. Here are several examples of unique situations and ways to focus on the positive and minimize the negative.

The Mature Nurse

Age discrimination is alive and well in the world we live in. Fortunately, it is at a minimum in nursing. However, it is still wise to keep your résumé age-neutral as much as possible. There are several ways to shift the reader's attention to your experience by eliminating information that would make it obvious how old or young you likely are. For example, if you list your first job as starting in 1975, or note that you graduated from nursing school or other postsecondary school that year, it is inevitable that the reader will mentally calculate your approximate age.

One way to minimize the age factor is to only go back 15–20 years with your employment history as outlined in the "Frequently Asked Questions" section at the end of this chapter. It is also advisable not to list the actual dates that you graduated from any educational programs. The exception, as noted in the "Education" section above, is if you are a new graduate nurse, regardless of your chronological age. (Today's new graduate nurses range from 20 to 70 years of age.)

If you still have an AOL email address, this suggests that you are over 40 or 50. Get a Gmail account even if you only use it for professional purposes.

Be sure to include any and all technology and social media skills such as working with electronic medical records (EMRs) and so on. This suggests someone who is current with all types of skills and not a technophobe. If you don't currently have any of these skills, start working to acquire them immediately.

The Newly Licensed Nurse

The big question is whether to list information related to major student clinical rotations on your résumé. If you are a new nurse who came to nursing school with little or no prior work experience, then the listing of clinical rotations on your résumé can provide relevant content. Just be sure to correctly categorize this experience as "Student Clinical Rotations," which will not be listed under "Work Experience." Recruiters are interested to see what types of facilities you did those rotations in (e.g., teaching hospital or community hospital). They are also interested to see if you did any of your rotations in a facility within their health care system.

If you have some prior health care work experience (worked as a nurse's aide, practical nurse, respiratory therapist, etc.), then it is generally not necessary to include content related to student clinical rotations. However, you can mention related information in your cover letter that might be of interest to a recruiter, such as the information mentioned in the above paragraph.

If you went to nursing school right out of high school, include work experience you had before or during nursing school, especially those positions pertinent to dealing with people, like restaurant server or sales clerk.

If you are a recent nursing school graduate (within the last 2 years), you should include your date of graduation from nursing school so that your status is clear.

It is neither necessary nor advisable to list your grade point average (GPA) on your résumé. Although you will hear some varying opinions about this, the vast majority of recruiters agree that GPA is not an indicator of a good clinical nurse and do not put much stock in it. Also, the information can work against you if it is less than a 4.0 and the reviewer does put stock into it, consciously or not. For example, a recruiter may be reviewing multiple résumés, several of which have included GPAs. The fact that one nurse has a higher or lower GPA than another can subconsciously impact the recruiter one way or the other, and not always in the way you would think. For example, a recruiter once told me that just because a nurse has a 4.0 GPA doesn't indicate that nurse is good clinically, and she might just be "book smart." So it really doesn't matter to her. She also noted that if a recruiter is considering more than one candidate and each listed their GPA on their resume, that might have subconscious influence on the recruiter in making a selection when, in this recruiter's belief, it really didn't offer valuable insight. It's better to leave that information off your resume.

If someone is interested in knowing what your GPA is, they will ask for it, and you can provide it. If you do opt to list it on your résumé for some reason, eliminate it once you are out of school for a year or more as it will no longer be relevant.

The Student Nurse

If you are a student nurse, you should include your anticipated date of graduation in the "Education" section of your résumé. That gives a prospective employer some idea of when you will be eligible for licensure. You can also list student clinical rotations completed to date, as a new graduate nurse would.

How to Develop and Update Your Résumé

Now that you've reviewed résumé writing basics, it's time to put what you've learned into action. The process of developing a good résumé may seem daunting, especially the first time you try to do it, but the effort will be well worth it. Once done, you only need to revise and update it periodically, a much easier task than creating it from scratch. Here are steps to create or revamp your résumé.

> Experienced nurse Agnes said, "I update my résumé as soon as I start a job and include the new position, so my résumé is updated and ready to go at a moment's notice."

Step 1. Gather Pertinent Information

Do some preliminary work by recording basic information about your education, licenses and certifications, and other key résumé elements. Make a list of all employers you've had, dates of employment, and title(s) held.

Step 2. Write It All Down

Create one worksheet for each employer and position and jot down *everything* you can think of that you did while employed there. This is a preliminary phase, so record it all. You can weed through it later. Do the same for professional association involvement and volunteer and community work if applicable. Once you've done all of this, put the information aside and go back to it several times over the next few days to add information as it comes to you. It will take some time to recall everything.

Step 3. Seek Input from Others

It's a good idea to ask a spouse, coworker, supervisor, or friend to help you remember some of the more significant things you did while in a particular job. We are notorious for forgetting, overlooking, and minimizing things that we've done!

For example, when I was developing my first professional résumé years ago, I drafted something based on my recollection of what I had done in each position I'd had up until then. For the position at the medical weight-control center, I had listed some basic things related to my day-to-day responsibilities. I asked my husband to look it over and tell me what he thought. Related to that position, he said, "What about the fact that you opened a new center for them, researched the demographics, oversaw renovations on the space, hired and trained all the staff, and built the business up?" I was startled when I heard him say it that way because, not only had I actually forgotten about all that, but it sounded so impressive when he said it! Sometimes we need input from others to appreciate how much we do.

Step 4. Choose a Format and Lay It Out

Once you have gathered the pertinent information and feel you have developed a comprehensive listing of accomplishments and experiences, choose the résumé format that is best for you. Start to lay out your résumé according to the samples at the end of this chapter. Choose information from your worksheets that is most appropriate and significant (review "Résumé Content" section at the beginning of this chapter). Break the information down into bullet points, like sound bites, so that each conveys only one accomplishment, responsibility, or piece of information.

Step 5. Craft the Wording

Now start to work on the wording of the information after each bullet point. Choose an action verb to begin each statement when possible. Truncate and shorten the statements so that each word has impact. Remember: Each bullet point should be one sentence or statement and ideally on one or two lines maximum. If it gets longer than that, you probably need to edit it down (review "Layout and Writing Style" section). Ask yourself: Can I say it better? Can I say it in a more powerful, proactive way? Can I be more concise? Can I be clearer?

Step 6. Let It Rest, Then Edit

Once you've done this, set it aside for a day or so if possible. When you come back to it, do more editing. Eliminate anything that is routine, redundant, irrelevant, old, or uninteresting. Repeat this process until you are satisfied with the content and the wording. It is common to do several edits before coming up with a final draft. Think of a good cook boiling down the juices and broth to make a rich sauce.

Step 7. Go Over It with a Fine-Toothed Comb

Look your résumé over for consistent layout and to check for spelling, grammar, and punctuation errors. It is very easy to miss errors on a document you have looked at repeatedly. Remember, your résumé has to be picture perfect. Don't rely on the spell-check and grammar feature on your computer. It is also good to have someone else, or a few people, look it over to make sure it is free of errors and also clear, concise, and complete.

Frequently Asked Questions

Q: *Should I tailor my résumé to fit each job I apply for?*

A: Generally speaking, no. That is not practical or necessary for the majority of nursing positions. For the most part, you should be able to develop one good, comprehensive résumé that will be applicable to most situations. Your cover letter is the place to customize; here you can mention specific elements of your background that relate to a particular position (see chapter 6). Of course there are always exceptions.

Q: *What if I work for a staffing or travel nurse agency—should I list every hospital I've worked at?*

A: No. Since you were not an employee of any of the hospitals, you would simply list the name of the agency you worked for. And since some nurses work for more than one agency at a time, it is not even necessary to list each agency. Rather, in place of an employer's name, use the generic title "Travel Nurse" or "Agency Nurse" (see résumé sample 1 at end of chapter).

Q: *What if I've worked for two or more employers at the same time—how do I list that?*

A: Simply list all positions as you would any others, listing the most significant one first. The résumé reader will likely note the date overlap. Many nurses have had more than one position at a time, myself included, so this is not unusual. A past employer told me that this was one of the reasons why he hired me for a management position. He figured that if I could juggle two jobs at one time I could probably handle anything that came my way.

Q: *How far back should I go in listing my experience?*

A: There is no hard-and-fast rule here. Most prospective employers agree that they are only interested in the last 15–20 years of steady employment history. That does not mean that you should only list employment back to that point. Besides, some people have been at the same place of employment for longer for that! Do go back a reasonable period of time, realizing that things you did more than 20 years ago have minimal relevance. If you had significant work experience prior to then that is different from what you have done in the last 15–20 years, you could add an explanatory sentence at the end of your "Work Experience" section. For example, if you have worked primarily in education or nonclinical positions for the last 20 years, and want to indicate that you have a solid clinical foundation, you could add a sentence at the end of the section such as, "Prior to this, had significant clinical experience in several major medical centers."

If your last 15–20 years of employment have been primarily clinical, it is not necessary to add that additional statement. If you have older work experience that is directly related to a job you are applying for, you can mention that in your cover letter.

Note: If you have been out of the workforce for a significant period of time (7–8 or more years), list your last several jobs, even if they were more than 10–15 years ago, to show some employment history.

Q: *Should I include nonnursing work experience?*

A: Definitely! Years ago, nurses were told not to include other work experience on their résumé. However, that has changed. Nursing, and nurses themselves, are more diverse than ever today. Many individuals are coming into nursing as a second or third career, and that prior work experience is both interesting and relevant.

Q: *Do I have to list every job, even the ones I stayed at for only a few weeks or months? In other words, is it OK to eliminate some things?*

A: That depends on how long you were at a particular job and why you left. If you had a job for a very short period of time, say a few weeks, and left because the job wasn't a good fit for you, you might opt not to include that on your résumé. If you left a job for any reason during an orientation period, you do not necessarily need to list that since employment is generally considered "conditional" during that time. If you were at a job for several months or more, then it becomes risky to eliminate it. Not only will there appear to be a gap in your employment history (unless you had another job at the same time), but also there is more likelihood that your prospective employer will uncover this information through networking and reference checking. Use your judgment, but be cautious.

A word of caution: Some states have laws requiring full disclosure by licensed health care workers of past employment. These laws exist to facilitate a thorough background check and to protect the public. However, these laws apply more to an employment application, which is an official document, rather than to your résumé, which is a personal document.

Most Common Faults Observed by Résumé Readers

- Poor overall appearance (e.g., in paper, print, layout)
- Misspellings, bad grammar, poor punctuation
- Not mentioning accomplishments
- Print too small
- Too wordy
- Too long
- Too short, sparse (e.g., no detail provided, lacks content)
- Mentioning personal and other irrelevant information
- Lengthy and complex sentences, paragraphs, phrases
- Difficult to comprehend (e.g., too many acronyms, unclear language)
- Key category or information missing (e.g., education, licenses, and certifications)

Résumé Skills and Experience Inventory

This list is provided to remind you of your own experiences and to help you focus in on the type of specific experiences and accomplishments that should be listed on a résumé. These are only examples and constitute a partial list. There are many others.

Speaking and Teaching

- Presenting at grand rounds

- Developing and presenting in-services

- Providing patient and family teaching and counseling

- Conducting community education

- Acting as preceptor or mentor to new hires, new graduates, or both

- Working with students

- Development of teaching aides (e.g., brochures, booklets, videos)

Business and Managerial Work

- Taking charge or supervision even occasionally

- Promotions you received

- Working on the budget or schedule

- Involvement with special projects such as developing or updating policies and procedures, research, quality improvement

- Manuals or special forms developed

- Being part of new programs implemented

- Liaison with outside agencies

- Special committee or project work related to department start-up, reengineering, cost-cutting, reorganizing, installation of new computer system, and so on

- Participating in employer-sponsored health fairs, health screenings, and recruitment events

Committee Work

- Any special or standing committees that you sat on or chaired, such as discharge planning, quality improvement, recruitment and retention, safety, and so on (committees can be unit-specific, nursing department, or facility-wide)

(continued)

Clinical Skills
- Any special skills (beyond the routine) that you developed proficiency in such as chemotherapy, ventilator management, ostomy and wound care, diabetic teaching, and so on

Technology
- Working with EMRs, proficiency in using PowerPoint and Google Drive, hosting Twitter chats, blog writing, moderating online professional SM groups, and so on

Q: *Should the education section be listed before or after my work experience? I've seen it done both ways.*

A: Either way is correct. However, a traditional résumé usually includes the education category after work experience. The curriculum vitae would list education at the beginning of the document after the summary if one were used (see chapter 6).

Q: *Do you recommend using a résumé writing service?*

A: I don't, for several reasons. Just because someone provides résumé writing services, doesn't mean they necessarily produce effective résumés. Anyone with some computer skills can produce the document, but that does not mean that they know how to maximize your experiences on paper or even that they are up on current résumé writing standards. Many of these résumés have a vaguely generic quality to them and are often referred to as "canned résumés" by professional résumé readers. In other words, they have a certain formulaic look and feel to them. This is a turn-off to a recruiter or prospective employer. I have seen too many bland, boring, and ineffective nursing résumés written by so-called résumé writers who list nothing more than routine nursing duties in an outdated format. The only person who benefits from this is the résumé writer.

While résumé writing is intimidating to most, once you learn how to do it and take the time and make the effort to develop one, you empower yourself on many levels. No one will develop a better résumé for you than you yourself can. And, once you have a good basic résumé, keeping it updated is easy. I have worked with hundreds of nurses over the years to assist them in developing a powerful résumé for themselves. I frequently heard, "It wasn't as hard as I thought it would be once I sat down to do it."

That being said, I realize that some people will still want or need the help of another person with résumé development and writing. In that case, it would be ideal to work with a nursing career coach or career counselor familiar with the full scope of what nurses do, as well as one who is up on current résumé writing standards.

Q: *If I worked part time or per diem, do I have to note that?*

A: No. List the position as usual, but it is not necessary to mention your status on your résumé. You can mention it if it comes up in conversation, or if you are asked.

Q: *If I've been out of the workforce for a while, how do I indicate that, or account for my time on my résumé?*

A: You don't. You can address that in your cover letter (see chapter 6).

Q: *Should I include my social media links on my résumé?*

A: It depends. Since LI has become a key self-marketing and networking site, it is common to include this link in your résumé or CV heading, but only if your LI profile is up to date. Other SM links and handles such as those for Twitter and Facebook can be listed in a separate section toward the end of your resume under the heading "Social Media" (see examples). But this is optional and should be included only if the content of your accounts would add value to your professional profile and not detract from it. On the plus side, listing this information can convey that you are savvy with contemporary communication tools.

Q: *I'm confused; why is there so much differing information out there about what should and shouldn't be on a résumé?*

A: There are several reasons for that. Some people who casually dole out career advice are regurgitating outdated information based on what they've seen and heard or what they believe to be true. They are often not career management specialists and have done no research or have no actual career management experience to draw from. They are also not in touch with those who actually hire and promote. Always consider the source when getting career advice.

Another reason is that there are some differing opinions and preferences about certain résumé details. For example, some recruiters might advise that you include an objective on your résumé because that is what they are accustomed to or what they prefer. However, most will tell you that it is neither necessary nor advisable for the reasons I have stated. The information and advice in this book is a synopsis of what the vast majority of career management experts, recruiters, and prospective employers have to say about career development, including résumé writing.

We'll continue our discussion of résumés and CVs in chapter 6.

Action Verbs for Your Résumé

Accomplished	Counseled	Headed
Achieved	Created	Identified
Acted	Decreased	Implemented
Adapted	Delivered	Improved
Administrated	Demonstrated	Increased
Adopted	Designed	Influenced
Advanced	Developed	Initiated
Advised	Devised	Innovated
Arranged	Directed	Inspired
Assimilated	Edited	Instituted
Attained	Educated	Instructed
Augmented	Eliminated	Integrated
Authored	Empowered	Interfaced
Built	Enforced	Interviewed
Chaired	Established	Introduced
Coached	Exceeded	Launched
Collaborated	Excelled	Lectured
Communicated	Executed	Led
Completed	Expedited	Liaised
Composed	Facilitated	Lowered
Conceived	Formulated	Maintained
Conducted	Fostered	Managed
Consolidated	Founded	Marketed
Consulted	Furthered	Mediated
Contributed	Generated	Mentored
Controlled	Guided	Met
Coordinated	Handled	Motivated

Negotiated	Progressed	Secured
Operated	Promoted	Selected
Optimized	Proposed	Served as
Orchestrated	Provided	Specialized
Organized	Published	Started
Originated	Ran	Strategized
Overhauled	Reduced	Streamlined
Oversaw	Rejuvenated	Strengthened
Paved	Renegotiated	Structured
Performed	Reorganized	Succeeded
Persuaded	Represented	Supervised
Piloted	Researched	Surpassed
Pioneered	Resolved	Taught
Planned	Restored	Trained
Practiced	Restructured	Transformed
Prepared	Revised	Translated
Presented	Revitalized	Unified
Presided	Revolutionized	Updated
Prevented	Scheduled	Upgraded
Produced	Screened	Wrote

Sample 1: Chronological Format
©Donna Cardillo. Reprinted with permission.

JANICE SMITH, RN, BSN
45 Lane Avenue Smithville, New Jersey 00090
(908) 555-2222
jsmith@net.net

SUMMARY

RN with diverse clinical and managerial experience in critical care and long term care settings. Excellent training skills. Possess positive, can-do attitude. Considered a team player and self-starter.

EXPERIENCE

SMITHVILLE GENERAL HOSPITAL, Smithville, NJ　　　　　　2012-Present
Clinical Manager, Telemetry Unit

- Clinical and administrative responsibility for 30-bed unit, including finances, personnel, and regulatory compliance
- Hired as a staff nurse, promoted to Clinical Manager after 8 months
- Designed and implemented a quality management program for unit
- Represent Department of Nursing on the following interdisciplinary committees: Infection Control; Utilization Management
- Frequent speaker for public outreach programs
- Act as preceptor to new hires

TOWNSHIP MEMORIAL HOSPITAL, Township, NJ　　　　　　2010-2011
Staff Nurse, Emergency/Out Patient Department

- Responsible for all facets of triage, emergency patient care, inpatient procedures, and minor surgery
- Directed outpatient clinics
- Administrated public screening programs
- Conducted orientation for new hires
- Coordinated department in-service
- Received perfect attendance award

TRAVEL NURSE　　　　　　2008-2010

- Worked with various healthcare travel agencies at temporary positions across the country from Hawaii to New York
- Developed proficiency in mechanical ventilator management
- Offered full-time positions at each facility
- Adapted to diverse work assignments including burn, oncology and pediatric units
- Assimilated easily, interpersonally, into each facility

UPSTATE LONG TERM CARE CENTER, Upstate, NJ   2003-2007
Staff Nurse, Sub-Acute Unit

- Responsible for all aspects of medical, rehabilitative and psychosocial needs of patient
- Assumed weekend charge position
- Supervised nurses aides and LPNs
- Proficient in EKG's and venipuncture
- Co-authored department policy and procedure manual

STATE HOSPITAL, Inner City, New Jersey   2001-2003
Staff Nurse, Medical/Surgical Unit

EDUCATION

Mytown University, Somewhere, New Jersey
  Currently pursuing Master of Science, Psychology
County College, County, New Jersey
  Bachelor of Science Degree, Healthcare Management
Township Memorial Hospital School of Nursing, Township, New Jersey
  Diploma, Nursing

LICENSES / CERTIFICATIONS

Licensed as Registered Nurse in New Jersey
Advanced Cardiac Life Support (ACLS), American Heart Association

PROFESSIONAL AFFILIATIONS

New Jersey State Nurses Association
American Nurses Association
Emergency Nurses Association
    Chair, Education Committee
Sigma, *Honor Society of Nursing*

AWARDS

MORE Award, North Carolina Nurses Association, Region 12
  For outstanding contributions and exemplary leadership

SPECIAL SKILLS

Fluent in German (speak, write, read), conversational in Spanish
Proficient in Word, Power Point, and Excel

Sample 2: Functional Format

©Donna Cardillo. Reprinted with permission.

JEANNE FARRELL, RN, MA
100 Meadowlands Parkway
Faraway, NC 00911
555-980-2386
jfrn@net.net

SUMMARY

RN with over 20 years of diverse experience in healthcare management, quality improvement, nursing education, and regulatory affairs. Dynamic speaker and trainer. Possess excellent ability to motivate, facilitate, and organize.

SPECIAL SKILLS

Speaking
 Frequent workshop presenter at nursing and healthcare conferences, professional association meetings, and community groups on quality of care and regulatory issues

Teaching / Training
 Trainer for ongoing employee/client relations program
 Taught gerontology certification course for local community college
 Volunteer lecturer for American Heart Association
 Provided customized educational services for long term care facilities to enhance operations

Writing
 Author of numerous published articles
 Created and was editor of nursing department newsletter
 Conducted peer review for continuing education articles and books

Management
 Broad management experience in acute, sub-acute, and long-term care settings
 Key team member in development of cardiac rehabilitative program
 Managed operating budgets up to $8 million

SELECTED ACCOMPLISHMENTS

- Featured speaker in The Joint Commission teleconference on revised long-term care standards
- Developed and implemented critical pathways for acute, sub-acute, and long-term care cases
- Created medical by-laws and updated physician credentialing process
- Revised physical restraint assessment program resulting in 15% decreased utilization
- Member of Magnet Steering Committee resulting in Magnet Award
- Received commendation status from The Joint Commission and orchestrated numerous deficiency-free Department of Health (DOH) surveys in both acute and long-term care settings

JEANNE FARRELL   Page 2

WORK EXPERIENCE

UNIVERSITY MEDICAL CENTER, Nursing Quality Improvement Coordinator......2010-2016
GGM CONSULTING, Healthcare Consultant 2014-2016
CITY COLLEGE, Instructor, Business and Community Development 2014
SUNNY SIDE NURSING HOME, Assistant Administrator/Director of Nursing 2010-2014
COLLEGE HOSPITAL, Head Nurse, ICU 2009-2010
UPTOWN HOSPITAL MEDICAL CENTER, Staff Nurse, Telemetry and Oncology..........2009

EDUCATION

MA Education, Unger University, Long Branch, NJ
BS Nursing, Saint Peter's College, Englewood Cliffs, NJ

SELECTED PUBLICATIONS

"QI: Everyone's Job," Nursing Spectrum/NurseWeek Nursewire, December 2005.
"Managing in Turbulent Times," Long Term Care Journal, November 2005.

PROFESSIONAL AFFILIATIONS

National Association for Healthcare Quality
North Carolina League for Nurses
   Board of Directors
National Association Directors of Nursing Administration in Long Term Care
American Nurses Association
North Carolina Nurses Association
   Mentor to student members
   Media Ace

LICENSES AND CERTIFICATIONS

Registered Nurse License: New Jersey, North Carolina
Certified Professional in Healthcare Quality (CPHQ) *National Assoc. for Healthcare Quality*
Certified Nurse Administrator (CNA) *American Nurses Credentialing Center*

COMMUNITY / VOLUNTEER WORK

YMCA Swim Instructor, adults and children
City Triathlon Club

Sample 3: Newly Licensed Nurse Résumé

Kurt Thomas, RN, ADN   H: 555-323-0000
1600 Paved Road   C: 555-331-9090
Inner City, CA 00502   kurt@net.net

SUMMARY
Newly Licensed Graduate RN with diverse clinical and work experience. Customer service oriented. Focused and motivated. Gets along well with coworkers, clients, and supervisors. Has an optimistic outlook and possesses a good sense of humor.

WORK EXPERIENCE
Inner City Hospital, Inner City, CA   2017-Present
Emergency Department Technician
Provided wide range of nursing support services in high volume Level II trauma center

Karl's Sporting Goods, Uptown, CA   2013-2016
Retail Sales Associate
Managed in-store and telephone orders, provided customer service, and instructed customers in safe equipment use

Inner City Community Pool, Inner City, CA   2012
Lifeguard

STUDENT CLINICAL ROTATIONS
Inner City Hospital...Medical-Surgical/Oncology
Mountain Community Hospital...Pediatrics
Center City Medical Center....................................Psychiatry/Maternal Child Health
Visiting Nurse Service Inner City..............................Community Health/Public Health
Veteran's Home...Long-Term Care

STUDENT EXTERNSHIP
Inner City Hospital, Inner City, CA   Summer 2017
Precepted clinical experience in medical/surgical intensive care unit

EDUCATION
California Community College, Los Angeles, CA
Associate Degree in Nursing   2018

LICENSES AND CERTIFICATIONS
California Registered Nurse License
Basic Life Support (BLS) Certification, American Heart Association

PROFESSIONAL AFFILIATIONS
Emergency Nurses Association
National Student Nurses Association

Chapter 6

Résumé Marketing, Cover Letters, CVs, and Portfolios

Although a traditional résumé is right for most nurses, there are certain circumstances where a curriculum vitae (CV) is more appropriate. While some folks use the terms interchangeably, a résumé and a CV are two entirely different documents and should not be confused.

A résumé, as discussed in chapter 5, is a one- to two-page document that highlights professional accomplishments, experiences, and credentials—a snapshot of your career. This is what most nurses need. In contrast, a CV is more comprehensive, includes much more information and detail, and is usually multiple pages long. It is generally reserved for doctoral degree–driven settings, such as higher education. It may also be appropriate for high-level administrative positions or in the literary world (e.g., editor, publisher), submitting work to be published in peer-reviewed journals, and being nominated for certain nursing awards and appointments. A CV might be right for some advanced practice nurses working in the clinical setting as well, although that is an individual decision. A CV attests to expertise and authority.

None of this means that if you have a doctoral degree or some of the above experience, you should shift to a CV. The format you use is determined more by the type of job you're applying for or the setting or specialty that you work within than your credentials. Not only does the average nurse not need a CV as a job search tool, but it can be a hindrance in a normal job search by providing too much information. It is considered overkill in your typical job situation. However, it is a good idea to keep detailed career information for your own records. The day may come when you need to develop a CV as you transition into one of these settings. We'll discuss that in the "Portfolio" section later in this chapter.

Because some people use the terms CV and résumé interchangeably, when someone asks you to send your CV, it doesn't necessarily mean they want an actual CV. Unless you're applying for the type of positions mentioned above, a traditional résumé is usually what they're looking for.

Unlike a résumé, a CV does not have a set format, but certain information is customarily provided. There are also some guidelines for CVs that differ from those for a résumé. Every CV is different, so craft one that best suits your background, unique experiences, and credentials. For those of you who will be using a CV, here are some of the typical categories and components used.

CV Components

Heading
Start with a heading that includes your name, major credential acronyms, address, phone number, and email address.

To Summarize or Not?
A summary statement, as described in chapter 5, is optional. But since a CV is generally rather long, a summary of the candidate's particular areas of expertise and interest along with strengths and personal characteristics will be a great help to the reader.

Education
Since CVs are used in industries where higher education is both a requirement and the norm, education is traditionally listed first in the body of the document. List each school in descending order by degree starting with postgraduate work, if applicable, and going back from there. Include the degree, institution name, any honors received, major and minor, and thesis or dissertation title and description. List internships, fellowships, and similar programs. Although dates of education can be omitted from a traditional résumé, it is customary to include them on a curriculum vitae.

With a master's thesis or doctoral dissertation, some prefer to list this as a separate category, which would include the thesis or dissertation title as well as a brief abstract (three to five sentences) discussing the content, focus, and methodology used. Including your advisor's name is optional.

Include academic achievements, such as leadership roles, grants, scholarships, awards, and recognitions as appropriate. Also mention academic affiliations, such as sororities, fraternities, and societies.

Professional Licenses and Certifications
Same as a résumé (see chapter 5).

Academic Teaching Experience
Include courses taught, courses developed and introduced, teaching interests, and a summary of teaching evaluations.

Publications and Writing
Include published works, such as journal and magazine articles, web articles, books, book chapters, and study guides. Also include work submissions and works in progress. If you have an extensive body of work, use the heading "Selected Publications," since pages and pages of publication listings lose their impact. Choose to list up to 20 published works, focusing on the most significant and recent. End with a summary statement, such as, "More than 100 published articles in 60 journals. Full listing is available upon request." When a CV is too long and cumbersome, the relevant information gets lost in a sea of words, credentials, details, and paper.

Presentations
List major presentations at conferences, conventions, and symposiums, including poster presentations. If you have an extensive number of presentations, as with publications, do list a substantial number of examples, but use the heading "Selected Presentations" and indicate the availability of a full listing upon request. There is only so much one reader can digest.

Professional Experience
It is customary to list current and past positions held along with titles and dates but not necessarily with descriptions like a résumé has. The format for listing employment history would be similar to a functional résumé listing (see chapter 5).

Professional Development
This might include conferences and workshops attended and other continuing education (CE), both live and online.

References
Unlike a résumé, a CV might list several professional references when the candidate is looking for a new position or seeking consulting or other work. If listing references, include name, title, and contact information. These references would ideally include deans, professors, administrators, and other high-level, high-profile colleagues.

Additional Categories
You might also include sections for:

- Research or research interests;
- Grants awarded;
- Administrative experience;
- Honors and awards;
- Consulting experience;
- Volunteer and community work;
- Professional association memberships and activities, including leadership roles; and
- Special skills, including languages spoken and computer and technical skills.

To recap, the résumé is a short summary, a snapshot of you. A CV is your portrait, your spec sheet.

Cover Letters
A well-written résumé or CV can attract the attention of prospective employers, but that's only part of the story. You also need a compelling cover letter when applying for a position or making a job inquiry. The two can be a powerful pair. In fact, some recruiters are more influenced by the cover letter than by the résumé itself. A cover letter actually speaks to the reader and helps you start the "sales" process. Even though many employers require an online application and/or résumé submission, there will still be opportunities to submit a hard copy or electronic cover letter so don't overlook this important self-marketing document. Here are some

tips for developing a cover letter that will grab the interest of the reader and make a great first impression.

While your résumé or CV will remain somewhat static throughout a job search process, your cover letter provides an opportunity to customize your application for each position. Here is where you reveal a bit of your personality and individuality. You can also highlight specific experiences, credentials, and personal characteristics that relate to this position. And you can mention your interest in, and familiarity with, that employer's company or facility, product, or service as applicable.

Always include a cover letter when sending a résumé or CV to a prospective employer, whether by mail, email, or fax, if it is your preliminary contact with them or if you are responding to a classified ad. The only exception would be if you were responding to an ad that specifically states, "No cover letters," or "Send résumé *only*," or there simply is no provision for one with an online submission. In this case, the company is probably in a preliminary screening phase and is only interested in what credentials and recent experience a candidate does or does not have. Including a cover letter in this situation might serve to irritate and annoy the prospective employer, and you risk bumping yourself out of the running for the position before you even have a chance.

It is not necessary to send a cover letter when emailing your résumé to a headhunter or agency representative that you have just had a lengthy phone conversation with. Nor is it necessary to bring a cover letter with you to a career fair or recruitment event where you will be distributing résumés and meeting prospective employers in person.

Let's take a closer look at what goes into making a dynamite cover letter.

The Format

Create a heading at the top of your cover letter, just as with your resume, that includes your name, credentials, and address as well as your email address and phone number.

Use a traditional business letter format that starts with the date followed by the recipient's name, title, facility, and address. If you don't have a specific person's name, address the letter to "Nurse Recruiter," "Human Resources Manager," or a department or position title mentioned in the classified ad.

Use a formal salutation, such as, "Dear Mr. Allen," or, "Dear Ms. Conrad." "Ms." is the universal form of address for a woman. We discussed methods of obtaining a contact person's name in chapter 4. If you don't have a specific person's name, you can address the letter to the entity in your address, such as "Dear Nurse Recruiter," or "Dear Human Resource Manager." As a last resort, you can use, "Dear Sir/Madam." Be sure to use both genders so as not to offend anyone. Avoid "To whom it may concern."

The Opening

The opening paragraph should immediately grab the reader's attention and be clear on why you are writing. If responding to a classified ad, state the position you are applying for (the company may be running multiple ads for various positions) along with the publication or website and date on which you saw the ad. You might start with something like, "I am enthusiastically applying for the utilization review nurse position advertised on the Nurse.com site on March 3."

If someone referred you to the person you are writing or recommended a particular position, mention that up front. Example: "Carl Howard from 3E recommended that I contact you about opportunities in the occupational health department."

Then go on to say something positive about the facility or the company as appropriate. For example, you might say, "I have always heard wonderful things about County General and would be proud to call myself a CG employee."

If you are applying for a position in sales, marketing, or training for a particular product, you might say something like, "Data Scan monitors are a superior product, and I'd love to help you spread the word."

If applying to work in a particular department or service, you might say, "Psychiatric services at County General have an outstanding reputation. I'd love to contribute to that."

The Body

The second paragraph should briefly summarize your qualifications and mention what unique skills and attributes you would bring to the position. This is your chance to let the reader know why you are well suited to the position, and why you are interested in it. This is also your opportunity to add relevant information that may not be on your résumé or that needs to be elaborated on, such as relevant classes attended, related volunteer work, and so on. Keep your comments brief and to the point.

The Close

End the letter on an upbeat note. Say something like, "I look forward to hearing from you so we can discuss our mutual interests further." You can include a statement about the best time and place to reach you if appropriate, such as, "Please feel free to contact me on my cell phone at 808-555-6333. Should you reach my voice mail, please leave your message and contact number, and I'll surely return your call."

End the letter with "Sincerely" (be sure to spell it correctly!) or "Yours Truly." Type your name several lines down, and sign the cover letter above your typed name.

Additional Tips

1. **Print your cover letter on the same stationary as your résumé.** If you have your résumé printed at a print shop, purchase extra sheets of matching paper to have available for cover letters. Be sure to create a heading at the top of the page that includes your name and address.

2. **Your cover letter must always be typed and never handwritten.** Keep it to one page.

3. **Use an assertive, confident tone throughout.** Rather than saying, "I hope you will find my experience appropriate," say something like, "I am confident that my experience and personality will make me an asset to the department."

4. **As with your résumé, the paper and print quality must be top-notch, and the document must be free of errors.** Don't rely on the grammar and spell-check feature on your computer. Have someone else look it over before sending.

5. **Use a conversational tone.** Don't use stilted language, such as, "Enclosed herewith please find my résumé." That is the language of legal documents, and I don't know anyone other than attorneys who can decipher it. Write as you speak. Make the tone upbeat and lively. (See examples at the end of this chapter.)

6. **Never use generic cover letters that you have mass-produced.** These are detected immediately and insult the reader, and will likely cause your paperwork to be tossed. You've got to personalize the cover letter when possible, and always customize it to the particular position.

A nurse actively seeking work showed me the worst example of a generic cover letter I ever saw. She had a pack of preprinted form letters addressed, "To whom it may concern," with varying dates, such as, "Spring 2017," "Fall 2017," and so on. This nurse had four versions with identical content but each for a different season. She had been using this "cover letter" to enclose with her résumé when responding to classified ads or randomly sending them to local hospitals. She wondered why she wasn't getting any responses. A résumé writing service had done these for the nurse so she would have a volume of cover letters for the entire year! I guess they thought her job search would take a long time. Ironically, her search *was* taking a long time, no doubt because of the generic letter.

Questions about Cover Letters

Q: *Classified ads often say they will only consider résumés that include salary history. How do I list that?*

A: Don't ever list your exact salary history on your résumé or in a cover letter. Instead, write something in your cover letter like, "Over the last 10 years I have been making a progressively increasing salary. I am currently earning in the mid-70s with benefits." This indicates that your total compensation package is worth more than $70,000 because your benefits have a dollar value, too. Remember: Don't mention salary *at all* unless an ad specifically requests it.

Q: *What if an ad says that I should include my salary requirements? How do I respond to that?*

A: First, understand that there is a difference between "salary history" and "salary requirements." Employers ask these questions in an effort to determine if salary will be a stumbling block in the hiring process. Since you know very little about the position specifics at this point in time, the best way to respond to this question in writing or on the phone, if asked, is to say something like, "At this point, my salary requirements are negotiable. I need to know more about the position scope and responsibilities. I'm confident that salary won't be an obstacle." You are simply giving the employer some assurance that you are a reasonable person and need more information.

Note: The issue of salary—when to bring it up, what to say when asked about it, and why you shouldn't bring it up at this phase of the job search—will be discussed at length in chapters 7 and 8.

Long before computers were the norm, many others and I had to plunk out a cover letter and résumé on an old fashioned typewriter. During one particular job search, I was sending out résumés and cover letters and never getting any response. I thought that was strange since I had never had difficulty finding a job in the past. I was discussing this with a friend, and she asked to see my résumé, so I showed it to her along with a copy of a recent cover letter I had sent out. She read it through and noted that I misspelled "sincerely" in my closing (I left out the second E). Spelling was never one of my strong points, and I foolishly did not have someone else look the letters over. Employers were probably thinking, How sincere can she be if she can't even spell the word correctly?

Q: *I've been out of the workforce for a while. How do I account for that on my résumé or cover letter? Should I even mention it?*

A: You should address a current, significant absence from the workforce in your cover letter, but not on your résumé. You can address this in the second paragraph of the letter by saying something like, "Although I have been on a recent hiatus from health care, I have kept current with issues and practice through contacts, associations, and continuing education."

Note: If you haven't taken steps to get up-to-date, you'll learn how to do that in chapter 8. It is not necessary to address past lapses in employment in a cover letter. This may come up on an interview, and you can address it then (see chapter 7).

Sending out Your Résumé or CV

While some employers will only accept online résumé and application submissions, on those occasions when you do have the opportunity to send a hard copy, it is preferable in most cases to mail your résumé or CV and cover letter via the US Postal Service (USPS). This is because a well-crafted and printed hard copy document can make a more powerful first impression than an online version, and first impressions do matter. To underscore this point, think of reading a book online versus having the book in your hands. The content is the same, but the actual book has weight to it, a certain feel and look, a unique character. Online, everything looks the same. Don't underestimate the power of tactile and visual senses in making a favorable first impression.

Another reason to send a hard copy résumé when you can is that you are more in control of what the receiver will get than you are with emails or online submissions. My experience has been that the US Postal Service is more reliable than email, although the latter can be quicker when time is of the essence.

While it is perfectly acceptable to fold a hard copy of the résumé and cover letter in thirds and mail them in a matching business size envelope, another approach would be to mail your unfolded résumé and cover letter in a white 9-inch by 12-inch envelope. Why? For starters, your submission will stand out from the others. An unfolded document makes a more professional presentation. Additionally, it will not automatically fold up on the recipient's desk, keeping its information visible and making it easier to handle. An unfolded document is also easier to file, photocopy, and electronically scan. And since an unfolded document is preferable for electronic scanning, yours will be ready for that, too.

Note: Be sure to use the extra postage required for this size envelope. If your résumé is returned to you 10 days later with "postage due" stamped on it or if it is delivered "postage due" to the recipient, it's all over for you. Also, type up a peel-off label for the address you are sending it to and for your return address. If using a business-size envelope, you can type the address directly on the envelope.

Enclose your business card (see chapter 10) if you have one. If sending a folded document, you can simply enclose the business card in the center. If sending unfolded documents, paperclip the card to the cover letter, or it may get lost in the envelope.

There are times when you will want or need to email your résumé to someone. For example, you may be responding to a classified ad that only provides an email address for contact—no address, no employer's name, or phone number. In that case, you have no choice but to email your résumé. Also, if you're working with a recruiter or prospective employer who wants to see your résumé quickly, it's OK to fax or email it to them if they request you do so. But it's still a good idea to follow that up with a hard copy.

When requested to email your résumé, unless specified, always ask, "Should I send my résumé as an attachment or in the body of the email?" It is never a good idea to send an attachment without permission or unless requested to do so. If someone wants it as an attachment, you can simply attach your computer file. If they want it in the body of the email, some reformatting may be required to keep it looking professional and the information easy to read.

Emailing your résumé can be tricky because some formatting characteristics can be lost or can shift in transmission, especially if the recipient has a different operating system than you do. Include a cover letter as a separate attachment or in the body of the email.

Remember: When mailing, faxing, or emailing your résumé or CV in response to a job opening, always include a cover letter printed on the same stationary as the résumé, except in the exclusions listed above.

Also remember: Your cover letter serves as your introduction and states your specific interest.

Posting Your Résumé on the Internet

It is common for job seekers to post their résumés online in the hopes that prospective employers or professional recruiters will find them and want to contact them. Many employers and recruiters search online résumé databanks to find job candidates. And since it is advisable to use every source available to you in a job search campaign, the Internet can give your search an extra reach.

Numerous web sites facilitate job searching and career management and allow you to post your résumé at no cost. While many career sites are general in nature, some are industry specific, such as those for nursing, health care technology, and the pharmaceutical industry. Some professional association websites offer this feature to their members. Each site has its own procedure to follow for posting and submitting information; there is generally a form to fill out to create your online résumé.

> Do not include a photograph of yourself when applying for a job. Some people think this will give them a competitive edge. However, this is considered inappropriate since one could suggest that prejudicial screening was done based on someone's looks, race, ethnicity, or age.

Most forms will request that you complete a keyword section. Since a prospective employer cannot possibly read all of the online résumés posted on any given site, they will search the database for keywords to help them find people with certain qualifications, credentials, skills, and attributes they are looking for. Therefore, you must carefully choose keywords that reflect your background, especially as they relate to a particular industry or specialty you are targeting. The right keywords can determine if your résumé is identified for further scrutiny or gets lost in cyberspace.

Likewise, when submitting an online application or résumé, many employers now use applicant tracking system (ATS) software to search for specific keywords and criteria. Rather than being screened by humans as in the past, many larger companies and health care systems now use computer programs to rank applications based on how well they meet the job criteria.

When choosing keywords, think of words or phrases that a prospective employer might search for. Read classified ads, both print and online, and notice the words and terms that are commonly listed in the type of position you are seeking.

While industry jargon and undefined abbreviations would not normally be used in a paper résumé, they are both necessary and useful in an online résumé where keyword searches are conducted. Be sure to use only common and universally recognized abbreviations, such as ACLS, NICU, OSHA, and PACU. Since you don't know for certain which words or acronyms each employer is searching for you might use both, such as: Emergency Department—ED. Note that the full name and acronym are separated by a dash with a space before and after it so that both will be picked up by the ATS program.

Following are some keyword and key phrase examples:

- Credential keywords might include: RN, BSN, CPR certified, ACLS, CPHQ (Certified Professional in Healthcare Quality), IV certified, and MS Healthcare Management.

- Since there are so many different credential acronyms for nurse practitioners (PNP, APRN, CFNP), include the acronym but also use the key phrase, such as "nurse practitioner." You don't want to be overlooked just because the employer didn't search for your particular credential acronym.

- Experience keywords might include: critical care, pediatrics, chemotherapy administration, oncology, trauma, outside sales, telephone triage, poison control, case management, care management, quality improvement, phlebotomy, substance abuse, administration, management, education, clinical research, ventilator management, community outreach, managed care, and regulatory compliance.

- Skill keywords might include: public speaking, teaching, bilingual, Spanish, counseling, project management, verbal communication skills, written communication skills, training, program development, computer skills, social media, PowerPoint, EMR — electronic medical record (include name of EMR program), and interpersonal skills.

- Keywords for other important traits might include: detail-oriented, self-starter, high-energy, team player, creative, independent, willing to travel, willing to relocate, dynamic, flexible, and highly motivated.

- Use short and common phraseology, like "home infusion therapy" rather than looser phrasing like "intravenous therapy in a patient's home."

Some additional tips and information about posting your résumé online:

- Examine the online form, see what information and format is required, and then prepare your responses in a Word document and save it. Then you can cut and paste it into the online form. Creating a Word document first allows you to spell-check the content (online forms don't always allow you to do that). You'll also have a record of the content you sent and will be able to use that content again for another form rather than having to recreate the content each time you submit an online résumé.

- Some job sites allow you to conceal your identity so that you will not be recognized by your employer (or others) if they happen to search the database you are listed on. In this case, you would be indirectly contacted by interested parties, can see who the prospective employer or recruiter is, and then opt to respond or not to that inquiry. Some sites also allow you to list search exclusions so that if your employer were searching for a particular type of candidate, your résumé would not come up when searched by that employer. (Users of the database generally have to register and log on before searching and so would be known to the system.)

- Since some employers and recruiters will search only for new résumé postings, sometimes it can be beneficial to remove your résumé from a particular database and then resubmit it if it has been online for a while. Be sure to keep the information, including the contact information, current at all times.

Adapting Your Résumé for Scanning

Occasionally a prospective employer will advertise for, or request, a "scannable" résumé if they are not set up for online résumé submission. A scannable résumé is one that is adapted for electronic scanning which replicates the document for online storage. Usually, an employer will specify what is needed for the document to be scannable. The general rule of thumb is: no bolding of characters, no bullets, no folds in the document, 12-point type size, white paper, and black ink. Any format of résumé or CV can be adapted to become scannable. You don't need to change the layout or content of your résumé in any way. You simply need to eliminate the undesirable features, adjust the paper color and type size if necessary, and send the document unfolded if sending by post mail. It is *only* necessary to adapt your document for scanning if you have been specifically requested to do so.

Portfolios

A portfolio is another valuable professional tool. It is not a single document like the résumé or CV. Rather, it is a compilation of information and supporting documentation that chronicles your professional history and demonstrates your ongoing professional development.

A professional portfolio serves several purposes:

- It is a good way to keep important documents and records in one convenient and organized place.
- It maps the course of a nurse's professional life.
- It supports and enhances a résumé or CV.
- It can be used to market special skills and experiences (e.g., writing, teaching, management).
- It serves as a tool for nurses to assess their practice and skills and plan for the future.
- It is a way of documenting what you do.

While it is not necessary to bring a portfolio to a typical job interview unless asked, a portfolio may be requested for consideration of admission to graduate school and when applying for certain positions and promotions. In these cases, you would be advised what to include in your portfolio.

Some organizations use portfolios for annual evaluations and for clinical ladder programs. Some states have considered requiring nurses to keep a portfolio as a record of clinical competency and professional development for license renewal. Even if you aren't required to produce a portfolio for any of the above reasons, it is still something every nurse should consider developing. At the very least, a portfolio is a good way to keep professional documents, records, and information organized and to keep track of career specifics that go beyond your résumé or CV.

Start Simple when Putting Your Portfolio Together

Gather all your appropriate paperwork. Use a three-ring binder with plastic insert pages or a pocket folder for the material you want to include.

Categorize your information, and arrange it according to some of the topics that follow. An accordion folder can help you initially get your paperwork in order and serve to hold excess or backup documentation, such as individual CE certificates, since you would only put a listing of CE courses, not all the certificates, in a presentation portfolio. A portfolio should be arranged so that it could be presented to another professional for review if necessary.

The content of your portfolio may vary depending on the specific use. However, it is wise to accumulate all of the information below since you never know how you may want or need to use it in the future.

There are online programs available to organize this information as well.

Formal education. Compile diplomas, courses taken, and transcripts. Consider including a summary or abstract of any research projects done, including a thesis or dissertation. Include special papers and presentations.

Professional credentials. Make copies of your professional licenses and certifications, including skills certifications (e.g., CPR, IV) and specialty certifications. This is an easy way to keep track of renewal dates and keep everything together in one convenient spot.

Continuing education (CE). Keep an annual summary of all courses taken, not just clinical courses. Include programs provided by your employer as well as online and live classes you have taken. Be sure to include noncredit courses taken, certificate programs, and the like. Keep course certificates in your accordion folder for reference and for presentation if requested.

Evaluations. Keep copies of annual reviews and performance appraisals. You are entitled to them, and should make it your business to get them. And while you want to keep all of them for your personal records, include only favorable reviews in a portfolio you are presenting for employment or promotion unless specifically asked to do otherwise. Also include complimentary letters received from patients or clients.

References. Keep letters of reference and your supervisor's contact information. (See section on "References" below.)

Publications. Include a listing of all published articles whether online or in print. List related work, such as book chapters written, and the like.

Presentations. Document formal presentations you have given at conferences, meetings, and symposiums as well as grand rounds, community education, and in-services.

Samples of your work. Keep examples of teaching tools, flow sheets, forms, and any other education, marketing, or administrative tools and documents you have designed, developed, or written. Also include a sampling of items that demonstrate your writing style, such as articles, white papers, reports, or proposals.

Professional affiliations. List memberships, offices and positions held, committee work, and special projects and programs worked on.

Awards. Include awards and special recognition from employers, professional associations, community groups, and other agencies. This includes service awards and perfect attendance awards.

Other professional activities. Keep a record of interprofessional committees you have sat on and community projects you participated in, including public screening programs and health fairs. Document teaching and training activities including precepting new hires and working with students. Don't forget patient and family teaching activities. (See "Skills Inventory" in chapter 5.)

Work schedule. Keep track of how many hours you've worked in a particular job, as this can become an issue with relicensing in some states now and in the future. For example, some states require that you work a certain number of clinical hours or "hours in nursing" to be eligible for licensure renewal. You may also want to keep track of how many hours you engage in specialized activities, such as diabetic education or wound care, since that information may be required if you decide to pursue certification in these and other specialties.

Volunteer activities. List all volunteer activities, hours of service, and special projects.

Accomplishments. Keep a special section on important projects and programs that you initiated, administrated, managed, or were a key player in. Include media events, starting up new departments, and major reorganization projects that you were involved in.

Annual professional goals. Every nurse should set professional goals each year and then evaluate those goals annually. Goals might be related to education, experience, skills development, professional association involvement, certification, and clinical competencies. We'll discuss goal-setting more in chapter 10.

Because nurses are notorious for underestimating their own skills and taking their accomplishments for granted, I recommend designing a worksheet that you can complete annually for your own records. The worksheet could include various categories to help you reflect on your experiences. For example, you might have a section on "management experience" where you would list any charge or supervisory experience you had, as well as budgeting, scheduling, and human resource (HR) responsibilities. This type of review could also assist you in identifying transferable skills, something nurses are not always good at. This worksheet can also help when updating your résumé.

References

Personal and professional references have become more important than ever in a job search. Most employers wish to take every possible precaution to ensure that the person they are about to offer a job to is not only competent and reliable, but also of good moral character. Therefore, whom you choose to provide as a reference is important. But even more important is how you treat your references since this can make all the difference in the type of recommendation you get from them.

Prospective employers may request personal and/or professional references. If they don't specify, *ask*, because there is a difference between the two. Professional references are people you have worked with and for who can attest to your level of experience, work habits, and how you get along with peers, subordinates, and superiors. Think of someone you've had a good working relationship with. Obviously, that person should be fairly familiar with your work. Many employers prefer to speak to an immediate supervisor, if possible.

Personal references, on the other hand, are people who have known you outside of work through your community, neighborhood, religious groups, professional associations, clubs, and so on. These people can vouch for your character, personality, habits, and so on. The more power and prestige the reference has, the more credible the recommendation will be. For example, a religious leader, community leader, educator, or prominent person in health care or business is viewed favorably.

You may be asked to provide two to three references in each category.

Once you've identified the people you'd like to use, contact them and let them know you are launching a job search. Request their permission to list them as a reference and ask if they would give you a favorable reference if contacted by a prospective employer. This is important for several reasons. First, it is the courteous and considerate thing to do. Secondly, some people may not be comfortable providing a reference for you for a variety of reasons, in which case they will likely politely decline. It's better to know that up front than risk having a reference say less than favorable things about you to a prospective employer.

Good references are a valuable resource. Don't take them for granted. I have often been contacted over the years to be a personal or professional reference for former employees, colleagues, and friends. I am embarrassed when called about someone I know when I didn't even know they were looking for a job! I'm sure the caller can hear my hesitation. Likewise, I appreciate it when someone who has asked me to be a reference provides me with all of the necessary information about themselves and the position(s) they are applying for. It makes my life so much easier, and they are inclined to get a better, more accurate recommendation because I am more prepared. I have also been contacted by employers to provide a reference for people about whom I have very few good things to say. If these people had at least contacted me beforehand, I would have been better prepared to discuss their strengths and weaknesses or could have politely declined to act as a reference for them. Getting caught off guard is never a good thing.

When it comes time to actually provide the reference's name to a prospective employer, contact the reference and let them know what position(s) you're applying for. Discuss the important characteristics of the job so they can highlight these things if they receive a call. Remind your references of your more significant accomplishments. Remind professional references of your title and duties while working for or with them. You should also send your references a copy of your updated résumé. Not only is this a great way to network (e.g., it keeps you fresh in their mind—they may know someone looking to hire someone with your background), but it will also remind your references of your dates of employment, job titles, projects, duties, and so on. In other words, do everything you can to assist your references in giving you a top-notch recommendation! No one can remember everything about every person that ever worked for them or about everyone who asks them for a reference.

Follow-up is a must with references and yet is so often neglected by the job seeker. Keep in periodic touch with your references to let them know what's happening. If you know they were contacted for a particular job, let them know the outcome either way. Definitely let them know when you accept a position. Take time to formally thank them afterward with a note or letter for agreeing to be a reference even if they were never called. In other words, let your references know that you appreciate them and their willingness to help out. It is also a good idea to stay in touch with your references even when you are not looking for a job.

Letters of Reference

Mobility characterizes today's workplace, especially in the nursing community. It is not uncommon for nurses to change jobs every few years or so. So when you are asked for professional references from a particular job, it is entirely possible that the person you reported to, as well as other superiors, is no longer there. You may be able to track them down through networking but that is not always possible or practical. That's why it's a good idea to get a letter of reference from your immediate supervisor when you leave a job. This way, you'll have something to show a prospective employer in the event you or they cannot connect with your work references.

As a general rule, letters of reference are not required in a job search process except in the above situation. Therefore, it is not necessary or recommended to send out unsolicited letters of reference when applying for a job. Some prospective employers do not put much stock in them.

Abbreviated CV Sample

©Donna Cardillo. Reprinted with permission.

Manuel Hernandez, PhD, RN
200 Center Street
Philadelphia, PA 00070
500-555-0396
mhernandez@net.net

EDUCATION

PhD in Nursing, Regional University, Philadelphia, PA	2006

Dissertation: New Graduate Nurse Attrition: Causes and Cures

MSN, Regional University, Philadelphia, PA	2001

Major: Adult Health and Illness   Functional Minor: Education
Thesis: Dietary Impact of Type II Diabetes Occurrence in Hispanic Population of
Philadelphia's 3rd Ward

BSN with High Honors, Harbor University, Baltimore, MD	1996

ACADEMIC TEACHING EXPERIENCE

Professor of Nursing, County College	2007-present

Fundamentals of nursing, senior leadership practicum, community health

Acting Chairperson, Department of Nursing, Mid-State College	Spring 2006
Assistant Professor of Nursing, Mid-State College	2002-2005

Course and curriculum development in new BSN program

Instructor, College of Nursing, Downstate University	2001-2002

Lecture and clinical supervision related to "Nursing Process in Secondary Care"
Teaching/research interests: Shared governance, medical ethics, nursing leadership

PROFESSIONAL EXPERIENCE

Maryland County Hospital	Medical/Surgical Nursing	2000-2002
Carter Memorial Hospital	Medical/Surgical Nursing	1998-2000
Mid-State Army Hospital	U.S. Army Reserves, CCU, MICU	1996-1998

SELECTED PUBLICATIONS

Hernandez, C. & Waters, J. (2007). Second Career Nursing Students; Challenges and
Opportunities. *American Nurse Today,* 4(8), 60-64.

Hernandez, C. (2006). Shared Governance in Practice. *Nurse Leader,* 10(4), 24-28.

Hernandez, C. (2005). An Ethical Discussion about End of Life Care. *American Journal of Nursing,* 12(3), 8-16.

SELECTED PRESENTATIONS

"Using Leadership to Enhance Your Clinical Practice," Emergency Nurses Association
Leadership Conference, February 2007, Boston, MA

"How to Apply for the Magnet Award," New Jersey Nursing Convention, March, 2007,
Atlantic City, NJ

Sample Cover Letter

©Donna Cardillo. Reprinted with permission.

Sheila Watson, RN
45 Lane Avenue
Smithville, NJ 00090
908-333-5555
swatson@net.net

November 8, 20__

Harold Meyers, RN
Nurse Recruiter
Cantor Medical Center
55 Main Street
Wall, IL 00875

Dear Mr. Meyers,

I am enthusiastically applying for the position of Staff Nurse, Medical-Surgical Unit, as accessed on Monster.com November 7. I've met many nurses who work at Cantor Medical, and they all speak very highly of the facility and its management team. I would be proud to call myself a Cantor Nurse.

I am an RN with two years of medical-surgical experience currently working in a small community hospital. Working at Cantor, a teaching hospital, would expand my horizons and my opportunities. My good work ethic, passion for nursing, and readiness to take my career to the next level would make me an asset to the nursing team. Additionally, I am always working on professional development and am planning to enter a BSN program in the spring.

I look forward to meeting with you so that we can discuss our mutual interests further. You may contact me by phone or email as I will be checking both for messages regularly. Thank you in advance!

Sincerely,

Sheila Watson, RN

Sheila Watson, RN

Sample Newly Licensed Nurse Cover Letter
©Donna Cardillo. Reprinted with permission.

Carl Fuller, RN, BSN
45 Lane Avenue
Smithville, NJ 00090
908-555-2222
carfull@net.net

November 8, 20__

Harold Meyers, RN
Nurse Recruiter, Cantor Medical Center
55 Main Street
Wall, IL 00875

Dear Mr. Meyers,

I am a newly licensed nurse with his sights set on working at Cantor Medical Center. I did a pediatric rotation there while attending County College School of Nursing and was very impressed with everyone I met. It was easy to see why Cantor has a reputation for providing excellent nursing care. I can't think of a better place to start my nursing career.

While working as an Emergency Medical Technician (EMT) on a volunteer ambulance service, I developed a keen interest in emergency room nursing and am most interested in opportunities in that department. However, I am open to other opportunities at CMC. I saw on your web site that you offer a special new graduate orientation program along with specialty internships. That was particularly appealing to me. My high energy, attention to detail, and readiness to roll up my sleeves and work hard would be an asset to your organization.

I would relish the opportunity to discuss with you how I can best contribute to Cantor's great reputation as well as what Cantor Medical Center has to offer a newly licensed nurse like me. Thank you for your consideration. I eagerly await your reply.

Yours truly,

Carl Fuller, RN, BSN

Carl Fuller, RN, BSN

Chapter 7

Interviewing

There was a time in nursing when you could pretty much just show up at a hospital, state that you were a nurse, and get hired almost on the spot. I always joke that the only question we were asked on a job interview in the old days was, "When can you start?" Of course those days are long gone, and nurses need to learn the fine art of self-marketing.

The thought of going on a job interview makes most people turn pale, get diaphoretic, and develop cold and clammy skin. The spotlight is on you during an interview, and most of us have difficulty talking about ourselves in a positive way. Nurses are generally not comfortable "selling" themselves, and that is exactly what you are doing on an interview: pointing out the benefits to the buyer, overcoming objections, and closing the sale. That's sales lingo, but it's exactly what you have to do.

The good news is that although individual interviewer style and format may vary, you can significantly improve your ability to interview well by learning and practicing the art and science of competitive interviewing. An interview is not simply a random question and answer session between two strangers. There is much more technique involved than most nurses realize. Once you understand the elements of an effective interview, learn to answer commonly asked questions, and get a little practice, you'll be able to interview with the best of them.

An interview is a time-honored ritual used for both parties to obtain further information. Each party has an objective and an ideal outcome. The interviewee's objective is twofold: to present yourself and your background in the best possible light and to get more information about the job, the company, and of course to ultimately get a job offer. You are evaluating a particular position and employer and trying to determine if the position offers the opportunities, circumstances, challenges, and compensation that you want and need. The interviewer's objective is to determine if you can do this job and do it well, if you are interested and excited about it, if there are any potential problems in your background, and to see if you will fit in and contribute to the employer's success. An interview is very much a two-way street.

It is important to understand that a job interview is a formal workplace situation and should be treated as such. It is not a casual social call. Therefore, you should dress your best, be on your best behavior at all times, conduct yourself professionally at every stage of the process, be well prepared, and keep your guard up at all times. More on all that in a moment.

Keep in mind that interview skills are not just for changing employers but would also be used when applying for a promotion or any new position within your current place of employment, being considered for a board position in a professional association, and possibly even being considered for a speaking engagement, political appointment, or award.

There are several different types of interviews, which we'll discuss a little later in the next chapter. For the moment, let's focus on the traditional hiring interview, where you meet face-to-face with the person or persons for whom you would be directly working.

Preparation

It is not always the best-qualified candidate but often the best-prepared candidate that lands a job. Likewise, if there are several equally qualified candidates for a job, it is likely the one that is best prepared for the interview that will be chosen. Preparation for a job interview is key to your success. The following tells you what you need to do in almost all interview situations.

Ask the Right Questions

When you are contacted to set up an interview, ask, "Who will be interviewing me?" Be sure to get the names and titles of everyone who will be interviewing you. You'll want to determine if this is a screening interview with a nurse recruiter or someone in human resources (HR) or if this is a hiring interview with a direct supervisor or manager. In some cases, more than one person will be interviewing you, either separately or as a group. It is important to know this going in so you won't be surprised. Don't be afraid to ask these questions. They are expected and they show you are intelligent and savvy about the interview process.

Agnes, a nurse recruiter, says, "Sometimes employers' schedules change without notice; the initial plan is to interview with HR and the manager separately but [you] might end up interviewing with both at the same time. The interviewee should be prepared and flexible if this occurs and not get freaked out. The interviewee's reaction to this unplanned situation will be observed. Remember the saying: it is not what happens to you so much as how you react to the situation!"

Do Your Homework

Before any interview, research the position, the specialty if applicable, and the employer (the facility, company, or agency). Research the employer by asking for some corporate literature to be sent to you ahead of time, such as an annual report or marketing material since all of this is not necessarily online. You can also offer to stop by and pick it up at an earlier date. If you do this, be sure to dress professionally and be courteous and professional to everyone you meet in the process. Just running in to pick something up doesn't mean that it's OK to show up in shorts or a sweat suit.

While you're at it, see if you can get a copy of the job description of the position for which you're applying. Also ask that any additional required paperwork, such as a job application if not online, be sent beforehand if possible. This way you can fill it out at your leisure and have one less thing to do on the big day.

Visit the employer's web site. Read their mission statement, press releases, and the like. Visit the prospective employee page (sometimes labeled "Work for Us").

Observe what, if anything, the web site says about the nursing staff and about their employees, benefits, philosophy, and so on. Note their accreditation status if applicable, the size of the facility or agency, how old the organization is, and so forth.

Do an Internet search for additional information about the employer and the person who will be interviewing you. Look for news stories and other related links and information. You never know what you'll turn up. View the LinkedIn and Twitter profile of the interviewer and follow them. This is not cyber-stalking but rather learning as much as you can beforehand. Then, during the interview, find subtle ways to mention some things you learned online. The interviewer will be impressed that you made the effort to do your homework. At the very least, you will be armed with more knowledge about the prospective employer and the interviewer(s).

Activate your network (ask around) to find anyone who now works for or has worked for the organization that you will be interviewing with. Ask them about the company and the department. Also, seek out information about the person you would be working directly for and the person who would be hiring you, if different. Try to find out about their management

Just as you might do an Internet search to see what turns up about a prospective employer and the interviewer, it is common for prospective employers to do an Internet search for your name to see what comes up. I recently heard from two recruiters who did an Internet search on two different job candidates and came up with information about prior arrests. If the information is out there, you need to know about it and be prepared to address it.

Also, everything you write on social media, a blog (yours or someone else's), your own home page, or anywhere online is searchable and can influence a prospective employer both positively and negatively. And since it is important to have a positive professional online presence, trying to hide your identity does not serve any useful purpose and does not protect your identity as some believe.

Some employers will go to specific popular sites and search for any posts by you. Search for your own name online and on various sites you contribute to, to see what comes up. Post responsibly. Always consider how what you write might affect you at a later time. This also applies to photos you post (avoid provocative poses and dress, holding alcoholic beverages including large red plastic cups, etc.). Of course you can adjust your account privacy settings to limit access, but then you miss out on the full professional benefits of social media networking. And nothing is really "private" online anyway.

style, their reputation, and their particular likes and dislikes in the workplace. Even if you want to keep your job search confidential, you can confide in a few close friends or family members and ask them to keep your name out of it when making inquiries.

To learn more about the specialty in general as well as the particular position you're applying for, do some informational interviewing with others in a similar position in a similar work setting (refer to chapter 3).

Scout Out the Location

Be sure you know the exact location of the interview and how to get there. For example, make a dry run beforehand, if necessary, during the same time of day as your interview appointment to observe traffic volume.

I was once in a downtown area store when a young woman came running in frantically saying she had an interview at 23 Front Street (the street we were on) and none of the buildings had the number 23 on them. No one in the store could help her, no one had heard of the company she was looking for, and she did not bring the phone number of the interviewer with her. She was already late and totally panic struck. I don't know the outcome, but it couldn't have been good.

Bring Your Best Self

Take inventory of your strengths and assets. Write them down on an index card or two or on your phone. This way you can review them just before the interview so they'll be fresh in your mind. Review your résumé and background especially as it relates to this position. Be prepared to discuss similar types of work you have done, especially when applying for a position in a new specialty or work setting.

Rehearse answers to commonly asked and anticipated questions until you feel comfortable and confident. Consider role-playing the interview with a friend or family member or rehearsing your responses aloud in front of a mirror so as to also observe your facial expression and body language. Some nurses have gone on interviews for positions that they're not too interested in, just to get the interview practice before the real thing comes along.

Start getting yourself pumped up and positive before the interview, the day of and even before. Listen to motivational recordings, read motivational articles and books, and use positive self-talk. Use visualization to imagine your desired outcome. For example: Picture yourself looking and feeling confident and sharp, answering each anticipated question with ease, getting a great job offer, and generally going through the interview process with panache. Do all this for several days before if possible. Listen to something upbeat as you drive to the interview, such as a favorite audiobook or the theme song from the movie *Rocky*. These things will help you stay positive and focused; they really work!

What to Bring

Since you want to be well prepared for anything that might come up, bring extra copies of your résumé, business cards, and a small pad of paper if you wish to jot down notes and information and to have prepared questions written down. The extra résumés come in handy if the interviewer can't find the one that you previously sent (it happens!) or if you meet other key people while there who ask if you have an extra copy. All of this shines a positive light on you and shows that you are organized, that you plan ahead, and are well prepared. You can carry all of this in a professional folder.

> Force yourself to smile even before the interview so your brain starts to become more positive. Of course, you don't want to have a nervous smile plastered on your face, so try to smile naturally. Stand tall with shoulders back and head upright. You don't have to actually be confident to look and act confident. Take a few deep breaths and go for it!

Upon Arrival

Allow yourself more than enough time to get there to account for any potential problems, such as traffic delays, getting lost, finding parking, and so on. (Make sure you have enough gas in the car and bring along the phone number of the person who will be interviewing you just in case!) You should arrive in enough time to be able to go into the restroom and check your appearance, have a few moments to compose yourself, and otherwise get yourself together. Check your hair and makeup or tie, dry your hands if your palms are sweaty, review your notes and your strengths and assets if necessary, and do one final round of positive self-talk or affirmations, such as, "I am an experienced, competent, and capable person."

If you're wearing an outer coat, take it off and carry it over your left arm so your right hand is free to shake hands. Unless you have been advised to come in early to fill out an application or other paperwork, wait until 10 or 15 minutes before your appointment time to announce your arrival to the receptionist. If you arrive very early, wait quietly in an inconspicuous place such as your car or an outside bench, allowing enough time to get yourself together and focused.

When you arrive, understand that you are being evaluated every step of the way, so be on your best behavior and be courteous to everyone you meet, including the parking lot attendant, receptionist, and security guard. People talk to other people. It's not uncommon for a manager to ask a receptionist, "What did you think of that candidate?" because how a person acts with ancillary staff can offer good insight to that person's true personality and character.

Elements of a Successful Interview
The Introduction
The first few seconds of any interview are critical. First impressions are made in as little as 3 seconds, and once they are in place, they are lasting and difficult to shake. Upon meeting the person who will be interviewing you, stand up (if seated), make immediate eye contact, smile naturally, and shake hands firmly (see chapter 10 for proper handshaking technique). This brief three-step process (handshake, eye contact, smile) can make or break an interview—it's that important. Extend your hand to shake even if the interviewer doesn't.

It is said that prospective employers make a preliminary decision within the first 2 minutes of meeting you as to whether or not they will likely hire you. That doesn't mean that the interviewer has decided whether or not they like you, but they do get a preliminary sense about who you are and whether or not you are someone who is confident, competent, credible, and personable. We'll discuss overall appearance and what to wear in chapter 8.

Once the introduction is made, the interviewer may ask if you had any trouble finding the place. Respond by saying something benign like, "None at all, thank you. The directions were great." Use this response regardless of the reality, even if the directions were terrible, or you got horribly lost. You don't want to offer any negatives into the interview process, especially not right in the beginning. And at this point, it really doesn't matter. The question is more of a polite opener rather than a query requiring a factual answer.

The Warm-Up

If the interviewer has come to lead you to the interview room, necessitating a brief walk together, you want to engage in small talk with them during this time. Small talk is that light, superficial banter we engage in when we meet people for the first time or see someone we know. While some people view small talk as a meaningless time waster, in reality it serves a very important social function and should not be ignored or downplayed. It allows people an opportunity to warm up to each other and get used to the sound of the other's voice before getting into more serious conversation. Take an active role in this, without chattering nonstop, rather than standing silently by and letting the interviewer do all the talking. You do want to let the interviewer set the tone for the conversation, but you don't want to be too passive, either. Here are some things you might say if the opportunity arises: "It's a lovely day out. I enjoyed the ride here," or "This is a beautiful building. When was it built?" Keep it simple and light.

The Opener

Once seated in the location where the interview will take place (allow the interviewer to indicate where you should sit), it's time to get down to the business of getting to know one another better and finding out if the job is right for you, and if you are the right candidate for the job. And while every interviewer has their own style and format, a typical first question is something such as, "Tell me about yourself."

This type of open-ended question is often asked simply to get you talking so the interviewer can get a sense of who you are and what your personality is like. Keep your response to this question light and brief, about two minutes in length, describing what you're doing now and what you've done in the recent past. Restrict your comments to professional work and activities and avoid personal disclosures. If you're not currently working or haven't worked in the recent past, you can talk about your career prior to that. Keep in mind that this is just an opening overview. There will be plenty of time to get into specifics later.

While the interviewer is listening to what you have to say, they will also be observing your nonverbal communication cues (body language, eye contact, facial expressions, hand gestures, etc.) throughout the interview. Some people are so nervous during an interview that they tend to clam up, get stiff, never smile, and speak in a monotone, which is not good. So here are some tips for conveying confidence, interest, intelligence, enthusiasm, honesty, and friendliness: Sit upright, leaning slightly forward. Don't sink into the chair. Make good eye contact throughout the interview without staring. Smile freely as appropriate, but not continuously. The use of hand gestures is good as long as those movements are low and close to your body. It is not necessary to clasp your hands in your lap as if you were in a grade school classroom. It is better to be a bit animated during the interview to show that you have some life and personality. However, if you are someone who gestures nervously in a distracting way, you may have to tone it down a bit. Speak in a clear, firm voice and let your personality shine through.

Remember to act confident, even if you don't feel confident.

The Needs Assessment

At a convenient time during the interview, as early as possible, you should ask the interviewer something like, "I'm interested to know what you see as an ideal candidate for this job." This is an important question for several reasons. First, it shows the interviewer that you are interested in what they want and need. Secondly, it will provide you with valuable information on how to best market yourself. You can't effectively sell yourself if you don't know what the interviewer is looking for. Otherwise, you might spend time and energy talking about your certifications and experience when what the interviewer really wants is someone who doesn't call in sick all the time because that's why they had to let the last person go. So ask the question, listen attentively to the answer, think about how you fit that "ideal," and find ways to get that message across to the interviewer.

For example, in answer to your question, the interviewer responds, "Well, we need someone with good communication skills because you will be interfacing with doctors, the public, and other department members." You might respond with, "That's great, because I pride myself on being able to communicate clearly and effectively with a wide range of different types of people."

Questions, Questions, and More Questions

As previously mentioned, an interview is a two-way street. You will certainly be expected to answer a certain number of questions, but you should also ask some questions other than those already mentioned above.

Ask Questions

Be prepared with a list of questions you want to ask about the job and the company. As mentioned, it is perfectly acceptable to carry a small notepad on which you have listed your questions. It's OK to make an occasional brief note during the interview (but bring your own pen rather than typing notes on your phone). Don't get carried away with this though. You want to be making eye contact and listening, not writing throughout the interview. Asking intelligent and relevant questions shows the interviewer that you are genuinely interested in the position and have taken time to research it and formulate questions.

In the early part of the interview, while you're getting to know one another, ask clarifying questions related specifically to job duties, responsibilities, size and scope of department, reporting mechanism, and so on. Here are some examples of early interview questions:

- What are you looking for in an ideal candidate for this job?
- Why is this position open?
- Whom would I be reporting to? What is the chain of command?
- What type of orientation or training program is provided?
- Describe the department staffing.
- Would I be required to work overtime or weekends, or take call?
- What type of support staff does the department have? (For example, volunteers, unit or department secretaries, aides.)

Later in the interview, once you have established rapport and have had an opportunity to sell yourself, ask more pointed questions such as:

- What are the biggest challenges the department faces right now?
- What problems or issues exist in the department that would need addressing in the first 2–3 months? (This is appropriate if applying for a supervisory or management position.)
- Where do you see the company or department going in the next few years?
- Are there opportunities for continuing education?

- Are there any opportunities for promotion from this position?
- How would you describe your management style? (Ask this when speaking with the person you would be reporting to.)
- What are the most important traits you look for in an employee or team member? (This is a more general question as opposed to the "ideal candidate" question which is more specific.)
- How long have you worked here? (This can be asked of anyone who interviews you.)
  - Follow with, "What do like most and least about working here?"

It is generally not appropriate to ask about salary and benefits on an initial interview. You can stop by the HR office for some benefits information (e.g., insurance, pension, tuition reimbursement) if you wish. We will talk more about the issue of salary later.

Sometimes, HR is the first stop in the interview process for signing forms, filling out background and reference check forms, and so on. Every company is different in this regard. If the HR professional offers information regarding established salary and benefits, then it is perfectly appropriate to discuss and ask questions of that person. However, all salary and benefits negotiations should be left for later in the interview process, as discussed in chapter 8.

Commonly Asked Interview Questions

While most recruiters and some prospective employers are experienced and skilled interviewers, other employers are not experienced at interviewing and are just as nervous as you are. Many will ask questions that they, themselves, have been asked on interviews or try to come up with something that they believe will give them insight into who you are. Below are some of the most frequently asked questions by interviewers along with advice on how to best answer them.

Why do you want this job?

This is a very important question and many job candidates answer it inappropriately. Your answer must specifically relate to the job in question. That is, the interviewer is interested to know what it is about this particular job or field that you are interested in. Do not respond by relating why you want to leave your current job, or that you are simply looking for "something different." An employer wants to know that you have some concept of the job responsibilities or of the industry and that you are deliberately looking to work there rather than throwing out multiple feelers hoping someone will bite. Your interview preparation work, previously discussed in this chapter, should provide information that will allow you to formulate an appropriate response to this question.

If you're applying for a position in a specialty or work setting that is different than what you've done in the past, the interviewer will be particularly interested to know why you are interested in pursuing this type of work. So, in answer to this question you might say something like, "I've done my own research, including speaking to several people that have been involved in this line of work. It has always sounded challenging and interesting to me, and I've decided it's something I'd like to do."

Why do you want to work for this company or facility?
Again, the answer must relate specifically to that company or facility. For example: "Liberty Medical has an excellent reputation in the industry, and I want to be part of this winning team." Do not respond by saying that the location is convenient. This is not a strong enough answer. The prospective employer wants to believe that you really want to work there because you think well of the place.

What are your long- and short-term goals?
Keep your answer brief and general. Think in terms of what the interviewer is interested in. For example, for a long-term goal, you could mention that you are planning to get back into school, if indeed you are.

Otherwise, state that you would like to develop expertise in this particular field or something similar. For a short-term goal, you might say that your short-term goal is to land this position!

What are your best and worst points?
Your response should indicate a best point that is significant, such as, "My outgoing personality," or, "My ability to get along with all types of people." Your worst point should be something that could be perceived

as a negative and a positive. Example: "My worst point is probably the fact that I am too much of a perfectionist and tend to want to keep reworking projects. However, I'm working on easing up on myself in that regard." Perfectionism can be negative, but it is really more of a positive. You have to state why it is a negative—in this case because you keep reworking things—and that you are working to improve it. Here's another "worst point" example: "I sometimes expect too much from the people I work with. However, I'm trying to temper my expectations and appreciate that everyone works at a different pace." Again, this is something that can be perceived as both positive and negative and ultimately will reflect positively on you. This is all part of the art and science of effective interviewing.

> When answering questions, think in terms of what the interviewer is interested in hearing about. That is, keep the responses business related for the most part. For instance, you might think that your best point is being a good parent, but this is not of particular interest to the interviewer. Remember, the employer is trying to determine if you are right for this job and if you can do this job.

Why do you want to leave your current job?
You may be asked this question if you are currently working. The best way to handle this is to say something like, "It's not that I'm looking to leave my current job, but this is something I have always wanted to do [or this is someplace I have always wanted to work], and when I heard about this opportunity, it sounded too good to pass up." Remember, you never want to introduce any potential negatives into a job interview. Any reason you might suggest for wanting to leave your current job is a potential negative and could open a can of worms.

The only exception to this would be if you have been notified that your position or department is being eliminated, in which case you could respond with, "I'm not looking to leave but as it turns out my department is being eliminated. Although I have always enjoyed working there, when I heard about this opportunity, I realized the timing was right for me to make my move."

Why did you leave your last job?

You may be asked this question if you are currently not working. Your response will depend on the circumstances of your leaving your last job.

- If you were downsized, laid off, or something similar beyond your control: "My position [or department] was eliminated, and there were very few other positions to go after. While I was happy working there, I saw this occurrence as an opportunity to pursue other areas that I have been interested in for some time. That's what brings me here today." The beauty of this response is that you have honestly stated the reason for your current unemployment while putting a positive spin on it, and you bring it right back to the job at hand. This is the art of good interviewing.

- If you have been out of the workforce for personal reasons, such as raising a family, or taking care of elderly parents or a sick relative, you can simply say, "There were issues in my family life [or personal life] that needed my full-time attention for a while. Circumstances are different now, and I am eager to get back into the workforce." An employee who is eager to work and not burned out is very desirable in today's marketplace.

- Use a similar response to address any gaps in your employment history, even if currently employed. For example, if asked why you had a 2-year gap in employment history several years ago, you could respond by saying something like, "I took a brief hiatus from work to tend to some family matters." You can reveal some specifics if you wish, but keep it light and superficial such as, "I was at home raising my children during that time," or, "I was caring for elderly parents." Be sure to add, "That is no longer an issue."

Regardless of the reason you actually left, you never want to say anything negative about a former company, facility, or supervisor. It does not reflect well on you. Be professional and discreet where former employers are concerned.

Be aware that some states have laws regarding disclosure of certain information by present and former health care employers when requested by prospective health care employers related to disciplinary action for poor or subpar clinical practice, substance abuse, and so on. This is one reason why it is best to be honest and up-front about these situations if they exist in your employment history. If you conceal something like this and the employer finds out about it later, you will almost definitely be disqualified from the position. However, if you disclose the situation and address it adequately, the prospective employer may be willing to hire you in spite of it, depending on the situation.

If you were let go due to problems of some sort, be honest but keep it very light and put a positive spin on it. Remember this is a job interview, not a confessional!

Example 1:
"I was let go from my previous job because I had excessive absences. I had a family challenge going on, and it was difficult for me to get into work every day. In retrospect, I should have taken a leave of absence rather than tried to juggle work and other pressing matters in my life. Let me assure you that the situation is now completely resolved, and I will never let that happen again."

Example 2:
"I was let go after self-reporting a medication error. Fortunately, there was no harm to my patient, but the facility has a strict policy about med errors. I was trying to do too many things at once that day and should have asked for help. I learned a very hard lesson from that experience, and I assure you that it will never happen again." Keep your facial expression neutral and steady. If you look like you're ready to burst out crying, it will scare the interviewer. Rehearse your response beforehand so you can deliver it calmly.

Example 3:
If you left your last job because you just couldn't take another day there for whatever reason, it is best to respond with something such as, "I was simply ready for a new challenge in my career and knew it would be difficult to launch a job search while working full time. I know it was a risky thing to do—quitting one job without having another one lined up—but I felt confident that I would find something suitable within a reasonable amount of time. Besides, this way I got to take a little time off to recharge my batteries so I can get started in my next position well rested." Say this with a smile on your face.

Where do you see yourself in 5 years?
The best response is something like, "I see myself doing [whatever you are applying for] but ideally in a position of increased responsibility." This is telling the interviewer that you have staying power, and while you would hope to be in a position of increased responsibility, as any person of average intelligence and motivation would be, you are not hell-bent on being in charge. Never respond with, "I see myself in your job." While many

people use this response and see it as clever, it is generally perceived to be rude and arrogant.

What type of salary are you looking for?

If you are asked this question at any time before or during the interview, prior to being made a job offer, respond by saying something like, "My salary requirements are negotiable. At this time I'm more interested in knowing if the job is right for me, and if I'm the right candidate for the job." If the interviewer pushes the issue, repeat the above and add, "We can discuss salary if we become mutually interested in working together. Besides, I don't know enough about the position and the responsibilities yet to have a realistic expectation."

The reality is that *you can't possibly have a salary requirement before you have more in-depth information about the position you are applying for*, such as if you have to do shift work or work weekends or holidays; whether there is any support staff; how big the department is in terms of number of employees, budget, volume of work; and so on. All of these make a difference in how much you would reasonably expect to make. Therefore, the discussion of money is pointless at the preliminary stages of an interview.

I'm sure some of you are thinking, "But I can't afford to make less than X amount of money, so why should I waste my time interviewing for the job if the salary is below what I want and need?" The answer is that you put yourself at a great disadvantage by mentioning a salary figure early on for several reasons. If you were to mention a figure that is below what the employer is offering, you can ruin your chances of getting top salary during the negotiation phase. Also, if you quote a figure well below what they traditionally pay, you may be perceived as not being at the level of experience they are looking for.

You can also hurt yourself by quoting a figure too high this early in the game and knocking yourself out of the running before you even have a chance to interview. That would be foolish on your part since, as already mentioned, there are many times that a job candidate comes in to interview for one job and is offered a better, higher-paying job afterward. Also, once an employer is sold on you and wants to hire you, you have some negotiation power, which you did not have early on. So even if your salary requirements are higher than what might be typically offered for this job, you are now in a better position to negotiate something that is more to your satisfaction. By contrast, you have no negotiation power early in the interview process. Once the employer is interested in you, everything changes.

In chapter 8 we'll discuss how to respond to illegal, situational, and abstract questions.

The Home Stretch

When the interview is wrapping up (i.e., it appears that the Q&A session is over), you've gotten all of your questions answered about the position, and the interviewer seems to be winding down, there are three additional questions you should ask:

1. **When might I expect to hear from you? Or, When do you antici-pate making a decision?**

   If the interviewer doesn't bring it up first, you need to ask. Typically, the interviewer, in response to your question, will give a timeframe anywhere from one week to three weeks. If they were to say, "Gee, I'm not really sure yet," you might respond, "How does 2 weeks sound?" The interviewer could say, "That sounds about right," or "Give me 3 weeks." You should never leave an interview without a timeframe for follow-up.

2. **Have you interviewed anyone else yet for this position?**

   If the response is, "No, you're the first one," move on to the next question.

   If the answer is "Yes" to the above, follow it with, "Where do I stand with the competition?" Say this in a light-hearted manner with a smile on your face, not in a confrontational way.

   Interviewers will likely answer in one of two ways. They'll either give you a very generalized, noncommittal response such as, "You're one of several qualified candidates I've seen so far," or they'll give you some actual comparative information that will give reasons. First, it shows that you are interested in the position, are assertive, and understand that you may be competing with others for this position. Secondly, if the interviewer is forthright with you, the information you obtain can be invaluable (see sidebar "Ask the Right Questions" on page 170 in this chapter).

   And last but not least...

3. **Do you have any reservations about me that I can clear up before I leave today?**

   I'm sure some of you are thinking, "Is she nuts? I could never say something like that—I don't have the nerve. Besides, what if they say that they *do* have reservations? Then what am I supposed to do?"

   As scary as it might seem to ask this question, it is actually one of the best things you can do to flush out and immediately address any reservations the interviewer may actually have about you before you leave the interview. Why? Because if the interviewer does have reservations about you, even small ones, and they are not addressed at the time of the interview, those reservations will loom larger and larger as time passes. Better to nip them in the bud.

Here's an example of why it's important to ask this question as well as how to address a specific objection:

Interviewee who does not have any direct experience related to the position they're applying for: "Do you have any reservations about me that I can address before I leave today?"

Interviewer: "You seem like a really nice person, but the truth is that I was hoping to find someone with more experience in this specialty."

Interviewee: "Look at it this way: You can train me to do the job exactly the way you want it done. I'm coming to you with no bad habits and no professional baggage." Of course, you would say this in a confident manner with a smile on your face.

The fact that the interviewer has some concerns about you is not a problem as long as you know what they are and can address them. As in the above example, don't expect the interviewer to think of this reason on their own.

ASK THE RIGHT QUESTIONS

Years ago, I interviewed for a position I wanted as a department director in a community hospital. I went on an initial interview, which seemed to go very well. The person who interviewed me, a hospital vice president, told me I would receive a phone call to come back for a second interview. I left feeling rather smug, assuming that I had the job and that the second interview was likely a formality. When I received the call to arrange the second interview, and to be sure my assumptions were correct, I asked several key questions. I first asked, "Who will be interviewing me this time?" I found out I would be interviewed by the same person as well as two other department directors that I would be working closely with. This would be done in a panel format (see chapter 8), meaning that I would meet with everyone at the same time. This information allowed me to mentally prepare.

I also asked another critical question, "Are you bringing anyone else in for a second interview?" I needed to know if this was a formality, or if I was still competing with other candidates. The VP responded, "Yes, we are bringing back another candidate." I obviously had jumped the gun assuming I was "it." So I asked another important question, "Where do I stand with the competition?" The interviewer was frank with me and responded, "To tell you the truth, you are both very similar in personality and experience, and frankly I'm having difficulty making up my mind between the two of you." Egads! I was competing with someone so similar to myself that he couldn't even make up his mind! After my shock wore off and I'd thanked him and gotten off the phone, I sprang into mental action.

For starters, I realized I had to be extra sharp and polished on the second interview. I was being evaluated by new people and still very much in a neck-and-neck race. Had I not known this, I believe I would have been somewhat complacent and let my guard down a bit assuming I had the job in the bag. Now I did just the opposite. I knew I had to find some way to distinguish myself from this other person who I did not know anything about other than she was perceived as "very similar" to me. So I racked my brain to see what I could come up with. Here's what happened.

At the end of the second interview, after all of the traditional things were discussed, the vice president asked me if I had anything else I wanted to add. This was my cue to tell them what I hoped would set me apart. I said, "I did want to mention that I've done some professional singing." Singing had nothing to do with the job (or so I thought), but I figured if they knew I could get up in front of strangers and sing, they would hopefully believe I could do anything. As it turned out, they got very excited about this stating, "We have an employee band, and they are desperate for a singer." They now looked more enthusiastic and interested than they had throughout the entire interview. Needless to say, I was hired into a job that was pivotal in my life and career on many levels. To this day I'm sure that they hired me as much because I could sing as for my other capabilities! All that mattered to me was that I got the job. Had I not asked those critical questions, I would not likely have shared that information, and who knows what would have happened. But since I knew exactly where I stood going in there and what I was up against—in other words I was well prepared—I got creative in my approach, and it paid off big dividends.

You have to counter the objection and turn it into a positive. Even if the interviewer says they have no reservations (whether or not that is a true statement), the important thing is that you asked the question.

Overcoming Objections

Here are some additional responses to common objections to be used *only* if they are brought up by the interviewer as a reservation:

No Experience

There are two approaches that you can use here, depending on the situation. If you are applying for something that will require some specialized training, such as utilization review or pharmaceutical research, and if the fact that you have no direct experience in that specialty becomes a stumbling block for the interviewer, you can take the tack previously mentioned that turns your inexperience into a positive thing:

"If you think I've got the right personality and attitude, you can always train me to do the job. You could hire someone else with experience but you can't change their attitude if it isn't what you're looking for."

However, in chapter 3 we discussed all the transferable skills that nurses have, and how we tend to downplay our abilities. So don't be so quick to say that you don't have experience in something or that you've never done something before. Rather, think of some way that you've done something similar in nursing. For example, if asked if you have any experience with case management, rather than saying no, you might say, "Although I've never had the title of case manager, I've been involved in the case management process by sitting on a discharge planning committee and having in-depth discussions with the case manager about my patients and their

---

IT'S ALL IN HOW YOU PRESENT YOURSELF

Krystyna had 15 years of clinical experience. She worked full-time in various clinical specialties and always had part-time side jobs in different settings and specialties, such as home infusion, occupational health, and quality improvement (QI) for a physician's office.

Krystyna relates, "While doing all that, I always kept an eye open for what was going on outside of the hospital but never had the guts to leave the 'secured place.' Being in a management position for over two years and dealing with cutting budgets, training nurses and techs to do more and more, and constantly pleasing the unsatisfied customers and miserable staff made me realize that I can do something else. I applied to an ad in a nursing magazine for medical research and was told that I had no experience. After I got off the phone, I thought about it and actually got mad. What did they mean I did not have any experience? I didn't directly do the same work but was involved in many areas of research while working in the hospital. So, out of frustration, I called them back, not thinking that would change their mind, but to tell them how much experience I actually had in that area. Much to my surprise, I was offered a job with one of the largest pharmaceutical companies in the world!"

postdischarge needs. I've become very familiar with the case management process." In other words, think in terms of what you can do, rather than what you can't do. Revisit the section on transferable skills in chapter 3 for some additional examples.

Out of Nursing for a While

If this objection comes up, the interviewer is concerned that you are not up to date with your knowledge, and they fear you may be generally out of touch with current practice. This relates to nonclinical positions, such as case management, telephone triage, or quality improvement (QI). (Note: An absence from clinical practice has different significance and requirements when applying for a direct patient care position. We'll discuss that situation specifically in chapter 9.)

You can say, "Let me assure you that I've kept current with issues by reading professional journals, taking continuing education courses, and staying active in my professional associations." (Hopefully you will have done some of these things in preparation for getting back into the job market.)

You can then add: "Look at it this way: I'm rested, fresh, and raring to go. I'm not the least bit burned out." This can sound great to someone who is working with staff members that are burned out and apathetic.

No Degree or Not a High Enough Degree

"I understand the importance of higher education, but you have to give me credit for all of the relevant experience I do have, not to mention my passion for this work. I can always go back to school and start working on that degree, which I would be willing to do if offered this job." That can sometimes be enough to get past the degree requirement. And getting back to school would be a good thing anyway.

Sporadic Work History

Acknowledge the situation by saying something like, "Over the last 10 years there were issues in my family life that periodically needed my full attention. That's all resolved now [or that's no longer an issue], and I'm ready and willing to get back on a full-time basis." You don't need to reveal any specifics. Much will depend on your demeanor and body language when you say this. If you appear nervous and avoid eye contact, it may concern the interviewer. If you seem confident and relaxed and have a smile on your face, the interviewer will hopefully accept you at your word.

Overqualified

If this objection comes up, the employer is concerned that you will not be challenged by the job, or that they cannot pay you what they think you should be making or what you've made in the past. You have to convince them otherwise by saying something like, "I understand how you might think that, but I see opportunity to learn and grow in this job. I'm interested and excited about it and am perfectly willing to work for the salary you're offering. Look at this way: you'll be getting good value for your money."

Remember, the fact that the employer has an objection is not the problem. You just have to convince them that whatever their concern is about you, it's not going to be a problem and may even be an asset for them.

Reframe the situation for them; assure them of your value, worth, interest, and commitment to the job and move forward.

The Finale

The interviewer will signal when the interview has come to an end, usually by standing up. At this time, again shake hands, make direct eye contact, and smile. Leave on a positive note by saying something upbeat such as, "It was a pleasure to meet you. Thank you for taking the time to talk with me. I am very interested in this position, and I look forward to hearing back from you!"

People tend to remember beginnings and endings so even if the interview didn't go great, you can leave a good impression by starting and ending strong.

Additional tip: Upon leaving, ask for corporate literature (annual report or other marketing material) to take with you if you don't already have it, and be sure to get the business card of each interviewer.

Frequently Asked Questions

Q: *Should I accept coffee if offered to appear sociable?*

A: You should never eat or drink anything on a traditional interview (exception: interview over a meal or a drink in a public place) even if the interviewer is doing so. Remember, this is not a social call. Besides, there is too much potential for disaster while wielding hot coffee.

Q: *Am I obligated to tell a prospective employer about a medical problem I have?*

A: According to the Americans with Disabilities Act, you are only obligated to mention a medical condition or disability if you will need special accommodation made on the job. We'll discuss special challenges related to disabilities in chapter 9.

Q: *What if I decide during the interview that this is not the right job for me?*

A: Proceed with the interview anyway, as if you were interested. As previously mentioned, there are many times that a different and often better job is offered afterwards. Also, the interview is an opportunity to establish a relationship with the employer and the interviewer, and you never know where that will lead now or in the future. Also, it's always a good idea to take a day to consider everything you learned about the job and to consider what's in it for you.

Q: *Should I carry a briefcase?*

A: It's better not to because then you have to worry about carting it around or accidentally leaving it somewhere. Besides, some prospective employers might consider it overkill. If you want to carry some extra copies of your résumé or similar things, use a professional-looking but unobtrusive folder or portfolio.

Q: *Is it OK to carry a small notebook and take notes?*

A: Yes, as previously noted, it is perfectly acceptable as long as you are not constantly writing. You want to stay engaged with the interviewer.

In chapter 8 we'll continue our discussion about interviewing, including what to wear, interview follow-up, salary negotiation, accepting a job offer, and more.

Chapter 8

Interviewing Two: The Sequel

Now that we've covered some interviewing basics, it's time to get more specific. Knowing how to respond to special questions, what to wear to an interview, how to handle various types of interviews, and how to properly follow up after an interview will make you feel more confident and in control. And if you use all the tips offered, you might find yourself in the enviable position of fielding job offers from several prospective employers. Then comes choosing the right offer, salary negotiation, and resigning from your current job. So, let's get started.

Other Types of Questions

In addition to the most commonly asked interview questions discussed in chapter 7, some interviewers may also ask a variety of other types of questions. These range from more in-depth or situational questions to the abstract. Following are several different types of questions you may encounter along with tips on how to handle each.

Situational Questions

This category of questions, also known as behavioral questions, usually starts with the phrase, "What would you do if...?" or, "Tell me about a time that..." You're given a hypothetical situation or problem or are asked to relate a real experience, asked how you would or did handle it, or how you would or did solve the problem. This type of question is sometimes asked in a more general way by stating, "Tell me about a problem you once experienced at work and how you solved it?" It might also be more specific such as, "Tell me about a difficult patient or client you once had. How did you handle the situation?" Understand that the interviewer is attempting to ascertain how you handle problems when they come up. In other words, are you rational, logical, and clear-thinking, or are you reactionary and defensive with a tendency to fly off the handle? Employers are wondering not only if prospective candidates have critical thinking skills, but if they apply and use critical thinking.

When asked this type of question, take a moment to compose your thoughts. Think in terms of what the interviewer is interested in hearing about. Keep your response simple, direct, and brief. Get right to the point and don't embellish. Remember the interviewer is looking for a logical thought process and a good outcome. Situational questions might also be used to evaluate a particular skill set. For example, "Tell me about a time that you had to plan a project or program at work or school. What were the steps involved and what was the outcome?"

When responding to a situational question about a real experience, you may want to employ what's known as the STAR method to keep your thoughts and your response organized and on target. STAR stands for:

- Situation: Describe a situation or problem
- Task: Discuss what needed to be done and why
- Action: Tell what specific actions or steps you took
- Results: Highlight outcomes, accomplishments, and so on

Abstract or Creative Questions

Some interviewers like to use indirect or more abstract questions that they believe will give them insight into the candidate's character or personality. Below are actual questions that nurses have been asked on job interviews along with suggested answers and tips. When choosing an answer to these and other abstract questions, remember to think in terms of what the employer is interested in hearing about. You might answer these questions differently if asked in a social situation. Stay focused on the purpose at hand.

Q: *What's your favorite book that you read in the last 6 months?*

A: As this is a job interview, choose a title of an appropriate book (no romance novels or politically controversial books please) you read recently or in the past. If you haven't read any books in the last six months, rather than revealing that, think of something you read in the past. Remember, the interviewer is trying to learn more about you, so saying, "I've been too busy to read," does not help your cause.

Q: *When you die, what do you want written on your tombstone?*

A: "Janet; she always got the job done." That one, or something similar, is sure to elicit a smile from the interviewer and a good feeling.

Q: *Imagine yourself getting an award—what award would it be?*

A: "Employee of the century."

Q: *Whom do you admire most?*

A: A nurse once asked me how she should have answered this question on a recent interview. I responded by asking, "How *did* you answer it?" She said, "My mother. She always had a zest for life and an appreciation of the little things that made life worthwhile, even while raising three kids and holding down a job." I couldn't top that answer. You can't go wrong with Mom!

Q: *Leave me with one word to remember you by.*

A: Here are some good responses: Dedicated, determined, passionate, enthusiastic.

Additional tips: It's OK to think for a few seconds before answering this type of question. Compose your thoughts and then speak. Be as natural and relaxed as possible with your response. Try to think of an answer that best serves your cause or purpose. This is something you get better at with some practice.

Illegal Questions

It is illegal to ask job candidates questions related to their religion, nationality, race, sexual orientation, gender, marital status, health status, age, disability, or whether or not they have children. This, however, does not prevent some unscrupulous prospective employers from asking the questions anyway. Here are some suggestions on how to handle the questions if they are asked.

A nurse once wrote to me in a state of despair having just come back from an interview where she was completely thrown by a situational question. She told me that the interviewer said to her, "A coworker comes up to you in the hallway at work and starts screaming at you about something. What would you do?" She felt at a complete loss as to how to respond to this question and believed that she blew the interview as a result. She wanted to know how she should have answered this question for future reference.

I first reminded this nurse of why this type of question is asked and what the interviewer's objective is: to ascertain how she handles problems when they come up.

I suggested that an appropriate answer would be something like, "I would respond in a calm manner by saying something like, 'You're clearly upset and I would be happy to discuss this further with you. But let's take it into the conference room so we don't disturb any of the patients or visitors.' I'd then start to walk toward the conference room in a way that included the other person." That answer probably would have satisfied the interviewer.

For example, an interviewer asks in a very friendly and nonchalant manner, "So, do you have kids?" Knowing this is an inappropriate question on an interview, you might reply in an even tone, "Does that have any bearing on the job?" You're letting the interviewer know, in a professional manner, that you don't intend to answer the question because you know it shouldn't be asked. They'll get the message and will hopefully move in another direction.

Beware of indirect questions meant to elicit the information without directly asking the question. For example, an interviewer might say, "I hate going to my kids' soccer games every weekend, how about you?" You could answer with a little humor and with a smile on your face by replying, "Are you asking if I hate to go to *your* kids' soccer games, too? Will that be a requirement of the job?" It will create a light moment, and the interviewer will see that you are savvy and sharp and not to be messed with.

Fortunately, the majority of interviewers are well versed in the laws regarding hiring and interviewing and are professional and ethical when it comes to screening and interviewing a job candidate. However, there are always those who try to circumvent the law and want to see what they can get away with. I only encountered this behavior on one interview in my career (see the next sidebar). Not surprisingly, it became quickly apparent to me that I did not want to work for this individual. I finished up the interview, did not bother to send a follow-up note in this case, and moved on.

I once interviewed for a medical sales position with a small entrepreneurial company. I first met with one of the co-owners of the company; all went well, and I was asked to meet the other owner. This second person was the scientific partner and clearly had less business sense overall. After our initial introduction and upon sitting down in his office, he began to frantically search his desk for my résumé. When it became apparent he wouldn't be able to readily find it, I pulled another copy out of my portfolio. He was visibly impressed at my preparedness. So far so good. Then, without looking up at me (acting as if he were focused on my résumé), he asked, "Are you married?" I paused for a moment, knowing this was an inappropriate question, but not having any experience with this sort of thing, took a brief moment to compose myself. It occurred to me that I had a wedding ring on my left hand so it would be easy to determine that I am married. I decided to respond, "Yes. Are you?" purposefully diverting the attention back to the interviewer. He seemed flustered by my counter question and in a nervous twitter responded, without ever looking at me, "Oh yes, I am." And then, without missing a beat, and still not making eye contact with me (I'm certain he knew that what he was doing was illegal and unethical), he then asked, "Do you have children?" Now I was getting miffed but didn't want to abruptly terminate the interview since I was rather interested in the position up to this point. So I took a deep breath and after a too long pause, replied, now in a rather curt tone of voice, "No, do you?" He replied that he did not either but still seemed unprepared for my counter question.

The interview deteriorated from there. The more time I spent with this person, the more I realized what an idiot he was. I knew I could never work for him or his company. So after the interview, I never bothered to send a follow-up note and never heard from them again, nor did they hear from me. The job, as I already knew, would involve some international travel. I'm sure this person was interested in my personal life to determine if he thought I'd be distracted or have split loyalties. Of course it was none of his business and had I been more experienced with this type of situation, I would have answered his questions in the way I suggest above, "Does that have anything to do with the job?"

What to Wear to an Interview

Your overall appearance is a critical part of a job interview. As previously mentioned, first impressions are made in as little as 3 seconds, and once they are in place they are powerful and lasting. So what can someone tell about you in 3 seconds? They can get a sense about you based on the image you project, including your clothes, accessories, grooming, posture, eye contact, and facial expressions. Countless studies have been done to indicate that each of us makes preliminary judgments and forms opinions about people based on overall appearance. That is why your appearance, including what you wear, is so critical on a job interview.

Remember: An interview is a formal business situation, not a casual meeting or a social call. Therefore you should look sharp, talk sharp, and act sharp. In any interview situation, even if you're not sure if you want the job, you want to be perceived as *one* of the best candidates for the job, if not *the* best candidate for the job.

Not only do you want to be viewed in the best possible light on every level, but you want to position yourself to be considered for the best job available (not always the one you're applying for) and the best compensation right from the beginning.

The traditional view for interview attire is that a woman wears a skirted business suit and a man a traditional business suit. Wearing a business suit to an interview shows a seriousness of purpose on your part, shows respect for the person you are interviewing with, and will make you feel more confident and look your professional best. Your clothes make a loud statement about who you are.

This does not mean that you will not be hired if you wear a dress or slacks or sports jacket and khaki pants. On the contrary, many people have interviewed in attire other than a business suit and been hired. But the better you dress, the more professionally and favorably you are viewed. While you may have heard that other attire is acceptable, a suit still makes the best impression. Besides, "acceptable" doesn't cut it in today's competitive job market. Even if you are of a younger generation and believe that casual dress is more the norm for your generation, you may be interviewed by someone from a different age group or simply someone who has a traditional view of interview attire. Conservative and traditional attire is a sure bet in most situations.

There are two exceptions to the business suit rule: If you are a woman who never wears skirts for whatever reason, then wear a pants suit. If you wear certain attire for religious reasons, that is also acceptable.

What color should you wear? It is always best to stay conservative on an initial interview until you get a better feel for the company and their culture. Safe, conservative colors for both sexes are navy, gray, and black.

Colors such as maroon or dark green are also acceptable for a woman. Avoid pastels. Red is considered an aggressive color, and while it might not typically be worn to an initial interview by a woman, I once wore a red suit to an interview for a sales position because I wanted to appear assertive and outgoing. It apparently worked because I was offered a job. Men should wear a white shirt and conservative tie.

Women should wear closed-toe pumps and hosiery (no bare legs) and men traditional oxfords and dark socks. Shoes should be polished and in good repair.

Your grooming should be impeccable. Hair should be neat and off your face. Keep your accessories simple and tasteful. Makeup and fragrances should be at a minimum. In fact, you are better off avoiding scents, since some people are allergic to or turned off by certain scents.

If you smoke, avoid smoking for a while prior to an interview. If you have a cigarette just before walking into an interview, nonsmokers can smell it immediately, and it is a turnoff to many people. Keep in mind that many employers have a no-smoking policy at work and many don't even hire smokers period. In the latter case, employees are required to sign an affidavit attesting to the fact that they do not smoke at all. If, after signing the form, it were discovered that that person did actually smoke, even on their own time, it could be grounds for immediate dismissal.

Interview Follow-up

As soon as you leave the interview and get out to your car, or as soon as you can that same day, send a very short text message or email to the interviewer to solidify the relationship. For example: "Great to meet you today. Thanks for your time. I look forward to hearing back from you soon! Have a wonderful evening." (Before you leave the interview, ask for business cards from each person who interviewed you so you have their names and contact information.)

An important but often ignored aspect of interview etiquette is sending a more formal thank-you or follow-up note after the interview via the US Postal Service (USPS). (This is in addition to the text or email mentioned above.) This note, which should be mailed no later than the day after the interview, sets you apart from the other candidates. It should be short and to the point. Thank the interviewer for the time spent, express your continued interest in the position, and briefly summarize what you would bring to the job (see example at the end of the chapter). If more than one person interviewed you, send a note to each person.

Your thank-you note should be typed on high quality stationery. Can the letter be handwritten? Although a few employers may say they find it more personal, many consider a handwritten note in this situation unsophisticated. How about an email thank you? That's only appropriate if you're applying to a technology company or have a short window of opportunity. For example, if you have a second interview with the same person the following day, a traditional thank-you letter won't have time to reach its destination. In that case, an email will serve the purpose. But of course, you can still send a traditional note to those whom you won't be seeing again. It's not necessary to send multiple thank-you notes to the same person for subsequent interviews. But a short text message or email after subsequent interviews such as, "Great seeing you again today. Looking forward to the next step!" is a good idea.

What if, after the interview, you've decided you don't want the job?

Don't be so quick to walk away. Send the thank-you note and proceed as if you do want it. There are many times that a different—often better—job is offered. Every interview is an opportunity. You never know what may happen. The better time to decline a job is when you're asked to interview again or are offered a position.

> If you're feeling nervous and rusty, get out and do some informational interviewing to feel more confident.

If you haven't heard anything from the employer within the designated time (the time should be mentioned, as discussed in chapter 7, when you ask "When might I expect to hear from you?" at the end), make a follow-up phone call to the person that interviewed you. Say something like, "Hello, Ms. Hawkins. My name is Carol Garfield. You may recall that I interviewed for the ICU staff nurse position about 2 weeks ago. I was wondering if you had made a decision yet?" Since the interviewer has likely interviewed several people for the position, they may not immediately recognize your name, so you might add something to jog their memory like, "I am the nurse that works in County General. You and I discussed XYZ College while I was there."

If Ms. Hawkins says she's still interviewing for the position, then you should ask, even if you already asked this on the original interview, "Do you have any reservations about me that I can clear up while you have me on the phone?" Why ask now and why ask again? Let's face it: If you were the ideal candidate, you'd probably have been offered a position already. If you open the door, they may be honest. It gives you an additional opportunity to sell yourself and overcome any perceived objections. Just asking the question shows you're a motivated, assertive person who's obviously interested in the job. If any objections are expressed, use the strategies and responses suggested in chapter 7.

On the other hand, if the interviewer has already filled the position, you might say, "I'm always working on my interview and self-marketing skills. I respect your opinion and wonder if you might give me some tips on how I could improve my presentation and marketability next time." Although it takes a bit of courage to ask this question, it can yield some invaluable feedback. Get something positive from the experience.

If you can't reach the interviewer by phone, you might try human resources (HR) or nurse recruitment to check on the status of the position. You can also try emailing the interviewer in this circumstance or sending a message on LinkedIn (LI). Unfortunately, some employers don't get back to all the people they interview. If you remain unsuccessful in reaching the parties involved after multiple attempts, you may have to regroup and move on. That's why it's always good to have a few irons in the fire.

The Right Approach for the Right Interview

So far we've focused primarily on the traditional hiring interview. That's the type in which you meet face-to-face with the person for whom you'll likely be working directly. But there are actually many different types of interviews, and each presents its own challenges. Here are a few common types and some tips to get the most out of the experience.

The Screening Interview

This is a preliminary procedure usually conducted by someone other than the individual for whom you'd be working, most likely someone from HR or a nurse recruiter. It might be done in person or by telephone. The purpose of a screening interview is to make sure job candidates meet certain minimum standards. It's also an opportunity to weed through the applicants and eliminate those who don't seem to have the "right stuff," either by background or personality.

Because this is only a preliminary interview, you don't have to elaborate on all of your work experience and special skills. You should answer the interviewer's (or interviewers') questions succinctly. There's no need to ramble or elaborate. Don't offer any additional information unless it's particularly relevant to the position. And while you don't have to give your whole sales pitch to this person—the hiring interview is still to come—you do have to impress the interviewer with your character, personality, attitude, and, if in person, appearance. Be friendly, courteous, and professional every step of the way.

Technically, it's not necessary to send a thank-you note after a screening interview, although it certainly doesn't hurt depending on the length and depth of the interview. It's an opportunity to express your interest in the job and demonstrate professionalism.

The Phone Interview

The telephone interview has become popular both as a screening tool and as a device to interview candidates at a distance. It presents a unique challenge for the job candidate because there's limited opportunity to convey strong nonverbal communication. The interviewer can't see you, they can only hear you.

Prepare for a phone interview beforehand just as you would a traditional interview. If this is not a screening interview, write down some points you want to make and any questions you want to ask.

When the time for the interview arrives, be sure to go to a quiet location with minimal distractions where you're not likely to be disturbed.

Remember, the other party can hear what's going on in the background, so if a radio is playing, a baby is crying, you're shuffling papers around, hitting computer keys, or smoking a cigarette, the interviewer will be able to hear it. Telephone receivers are very sound sensitive.

When it's time to talk, put a smile on your face even though the person on the other end can't see it. When you smile, there's something in your voice that conveys friendliness and confidence. Use an enthusiastic and assertive tone, and listen attentively. Speak slowly and clearly, taking time to enunciate your words. And even though the interviewer can't see you, *dress professionally*; research has demonstrated that people act more professionally when they are dressed the part, even on the telephone!

If the phone interview is something other than a preliminary screening interview, send a thank-you note afterward.

The Follow-up Interview

This is often one in a series of hiring interviews for a specific position. It might be done with the person who previously interviewed you or with different people. The purpose is to see how you fit in with the team and to get to know you better. Don't let down your guard or assume you have the job because you're being brought back: Dress and act as sharp as you did during the first interview. If possible, wear a different outfit for each visit. Be prepared for situational questions, such as, "What is the first thing you'd do as manager if you get this job?" or, "How would you handle this situation?"

Reminder: As discussed in chapter 7, be sure to ask if anyone else is being brought in for a second interview or if anyone else is also being considered for the position. If the answer is yes, ask, "Where do I stand with the competition?" *Remember, it is often the best-prepared candidate who gets the job.*

Send a thank-you note to anyone who interviewed you for the first time. While it is not necessary to send another formal typed note to the same person for subsequent interviews, a short email follow-up instead is appropriate, such as:

Dear Amad,

It was nice to see you again today. Thank you for setting up the interview with Allen and Fred. I enjoyed meeting them and further discussing the position.

We certainly had some lively discussion! I look forward to our next meeting.

Best Wishes,

Ayesha

The Panel Interview

This is when you're interviewed by more than one person in the same room at the same time. This is sometimes done as the preliminary interview in a series, or it might be the format for a subsequent interview. The panel might be various members of a particular department, or it might be several supervisors or managers if you're applying for a management position. That's why it's important to always ask beforehand who will be interviewing you. Reminder: Get the names and titles of those involved. That way, you'll be well prepared.

A panel interview can be intimidating, but it doesn't have to be if you're prepared. On entering the interview room, make eye contact with all the participants and shake each person's hand before and after the interview, even if you have to walk around a table to do so. Listen carefully to each person's name and repeat it after it is told to you. This will help you to remember it when you first hear it. If possible, address everyone by name during the interview. This is not absolutely necessary, so don't panic, however it will win you some points if you can manage to do it.

One person will likely take the lead during the interview and ask most of the questions, but be sure to direct your answers to and make eye contact with everyone in the room. Ask for each person's business card at the end of the interview, shake everyone's hand again, tell them it was a pleasure to meet with them, and thank them for their time. Send a follow-up note to each person.

The In-House Interview

This is an interview for a position other than your current one with the organization that you already work for. For example, you might currently be a clinical bedside nurse in a hospital and have decided to apply for a unit manager position or staff development job. Treat this type of interview as you would any other, even if you are already acquainted with the person who will be interviewing you. That is, apply for the position using a cover letter and submitting a résumé.

When it's time for the interview, try to make the appointment before or after your work hours or on your day off so that you are not distracted and can be more focused. It is ideal if you wear proper interview attire to the interview even if you have to change at work. Send a thank-you note and follow the described follow-up procedure.

The Dinner Interview

Interviews conducted over dinner are most common when applying for a management position or one in which you will be dealing with the public, such as a sales or marketing position. It gives both parties an opportunity to get to know each other in a less structured format. It's also an opportunity for the interviewer to better observe your social graces and your ability to handle yourself in a variety of situations.

To prepare, brush up on your dining etiquette beforehand, if necessary, by referring to appropriate books or articles. Follow the interviewer's (or interviewers') lead when ordering an appetizer, entrée, and so on. You don't have to order the same thing as them, but you should order something in the same general price range and of the same type. If the interviewer doesn't order an appetizer than you should forgo the appetizer as well.

Proceed with caution where alcoholic beverages are concerned. If the interviewer orders a glass of wine or beer, it would be appropriate for you to also order same—only if you wish—and only at a dinner interview, not at lunch. If you do order alcohol, stick to wine or beer (and only if the interviewer also orders the same), and sip your drink. Don't finish it. If you don't want an alcoholic beverage, it's fine to order a soft drink or water. One recruiter I spoke with is of the mind that a job candidate should not order any alcohol on an interview. Use your best judgment and always err on the side of caution.

Remember that it's still an interview—not a night out—so dress and act accordingly.

The Group Interview
This is the type where multiple candidates are interviewed as a group, often at a facility open house or open application event as well as for graduate school applicants. You can stand out from the crowd by being appropriately dressed, making good eye contact with the interviewer, and smiling as appropriate. Ask one or two questions when the opportunity presents itself, but don't dominate the session. Afterward, be sure to approach the interviewer(s), introduce yourself, and shake their hand. Obtain this person's business card, provide yours if you have one (you should!), and send a thank-you note, even for a graduate school interview. All of this will help distinguish you in a positive way.

The Impromptu Interview
This type of interview is conducted at career fairs or at on-site open-house events. There is usually a crowd present and a fair amount of noise and activity. Both the recruiter and the prospect are standing and conversing. An impromptu interview is brief and preliminary to give the recruiter a sense of whom they wish to speak with further after the event. Make a good first impression by being well dressed and well prepared with your résumé

and business card. Shake hands, make good eye contact, and smile. Present yourself as friendly, upbeat, personable, and enthusiastic. Since there is little time at these events to discuss specifics, convey interest in the employer's need and express your particular interests but remain open to further discussion and possible opportunities. In other words, keep an open mind. This approach is guaranteed to get you a call back.

There are some occasions when recruiters at these events have made arrangements to have more in-depth interviews with candidates that they are interested in. So, if you make a good impression and have the background that the recruiter is looking for, you just might be asked to sit down somewhere to talk further. It happens sometimes, so be prepared!

The Video Interview

This type of interview allows both parties to see and interact with one another regardless of geographic location. Skype or another program on your computer or phone would be required. If you don't have access to the right technology or aren't sure how to use it, find someone who does and have them help you install the necessary components on your computer, then do a practice session with them before the interview.

Prepare as you would for any interview. Dress in subdued colors, avoiding red, white, stripes, and patterns since these do not show well on video and certain patterns can create optical distortions on camera. Wait for the other party to finish speaking completely before responding. Listen attentively and use good nonverbal communication: sit upright, smile as appropriate, and make good "eye contact" with the camera. Focus on the recruiter's image and don't be distracted by your own image, which is usually shown on another screen or window. In this type of interview, hand gestures should be minimal since they can be distracting.

Juggling Job Offers

It's bound to happen at some point. You're going on multiple job interviews, trying to find just the right spot for your next career move. Things are going fairly well, and you've found several different positions that interest you. So far so good, right? But what if you get offered one job while waiting to hear from another that you prefer? Or what if you're offered a job before you've even interviewed for the position in which you're really interested? Learning professional strategies to juggle job offers will help you find the position that's right for you.

Scenario One

You've been on several interviews. Although all of the positions interest you, there's one in particular you're really excited about, and you hope you'll get an offer for it. In the meantime, you get an offer for another position. The pay is pretty good, and it's a good company. You can picture yourself working there, but you can't help but wonder about the other position. Should you say no to the offer and hold out for the position you really want? Or should you take the offer, knowing even though it may not be your ideal job, you'll feel more secure and can stop interviewing?

Strategy

There's a natural tendency to grab the first job offer that comes your way because it gives you a sense of security. However, the purpose of interviewing is to thoroughly explore your options and find a position that's a good move for you.

Tell the company that's making the offer you're interested in the position, but you're actively interviewing and need a little more time to consider your options. Some companies will take this better than others. You might ask, "May I have a few days to think it over?" Most employers are unwilling to wait very long for an answer. Understandably, they'll want to move on to the next candidate if you decide you don't want the job. They'll probably give you a timeframe to respond or ask you how much time you need. Negotiate for as much time as possible, but be reasonable. No employer will wait forever while you make up your mind.

Then contact the employer you're really interested in working for. Tell the company you've received another job offer, but you'd prefer to work for them. Because you have to make a decision about the other job offer within a reasonable period of time, ask what your prospects are with them. Even if your ideal employer is not yet ready to make a final decision, it's hoped the company will be honest with you about your chances of getting hired. At least you'll know where you stand and decide whether to wait or not.

Scenario Two

You've met with some prospective employers and still have some interesting interviews lined up. One upcoming interview sounds particularly intriguing, and you're looking forward to learning more about the position and the company. Before the interview occurs, you receive a job offer from another company. The offer is tempting, but you're dying to take a shot at the other position.

Strategy

As in the first scenario, let the employer who made the offer know you're actively interviewing and would like a little more time to consider all of your options. Call your ideal employer and tell them you've received another job offer. Let them know you're particularly interested in the position they advertise and ask if the interview can be moved up. You can advise them you'd like to see if the job might be a good fit for both parties before you make a decision about the other offer. Of course, if that isn't possible, then you may have to take your chances and let the first job go while you pursue the other.

Scenario Three

Another possibility is you receive two or more job offerings within the span of several days. It has happened! One of the jobs offered is your distinct preference, but the other job offers better salary, benefits, hours, or whatever.

Strategy

See if you can buy some time from the offering employers. Tell your preferred employer that you're most interested in this position but have been made another offer with a better salary, benefits, or whatever the factor is. Ask if there is any room for negotiation. Stress that you would prefer to work for them and would be able to easily make your decision if the offer could be matched or at least improved. You're at an advantage here, but don't flaunt it. Be honest with your preferred employer, and see if you can work things out.

How to Negotiate the Salary You Want

Unfortunately, it's impossible to negotiate salary in every position you go after. For example, when you apply for a clinical bedside position in a public health care facility, salaries are usually predetermined and pretty much set in stone. They're based on objective criteria, such as years of experience, degrees, certifications, shift differential, and so on. However, once you get into management, or in some cases, private health care facilities, and more nontraditional jobs, there is usually leeway to negotiate.

Here are the rules for successful salary negotiating.

Do Your Homework

Find out what the going salary is for a comparable position in your geographic area. Search online job databases, do an Internet search, or contact the state arm of a related national professional association for salary surveys or information. For example, if you are applying for a nurse educator's position in a hospital, contact your state chapter of the Association of Nursing Professional Development (ANPD) and find out if the chapter or the national office has done any salary surveys in the last 5 years.

Another effective way to find salary information is to network with others in the industry. While it's considered rude to ask someone how much they make, it's perfectly acceptable to ask, "What's a ballpark salary for a hospital-based nurse educator position in this geographic area?" If you can't find information on the same job in the same type of setting, look for something with similar responsibilities. This type of information can be obtained through routine informational interviewing, or you can simply conduct your own informal salary survey. In the latter case, promise to share your findings with those who offer you information.

Let Them Mention a Number First

Once you've been offered a job, try to get the prospective employer to quote a number or salary range first. In an employment situation, whoever mentions a salary figure first is at a disadvantage. So if you're asked what you think would be a fair salary, say something like, "How much have you budgeted for this position?" or, "How much were you paying the last person? Let's start there." Many employers will be upfront with this information. Then you can gauge what you have to work with.

Know Your Bottom Line

Be prepared ahead of time with a ballpark amount that you want that is based on your knowledge, research, and experience. Also know, what's the least amount you're willing to take? And since both salary and benefits make up your total compensation package, you have to look at the big picture; don't fixate solely on hourly rate or annual wages. Consider the total health care coverage package; does it include eyeglass and dental coverage? How much tuition reimbursement is offered? Does the employer have a 401(k) program with matched annual savings? Are you eligible for a pension? Everything has an associated dollar value.

Likewise, you have to consider the general working conditions and schedule as well as the type of work you will be doing. For example, how much vacation is allotted? I once spoke with a nurse who took a $6,000/year pay cut when she transitioned from the hospital to a law office working as a legal nurse consultant. However, she received more comprehensive health care benefits for herself and her family, and she got 7 weeks of paid vacation! That was worth more to her than the extra salary. Benefits can account for up to half of your total compensation package.

Ask for a Little More Money than You're Offered

There's usually a salary range, and people rarely offer the top amount. If your request is reasonable and the employer wants you and has the budget, you may get what you ask for. The worst that could happen is that your request gets turned down. But asking doesn't jeopardize your standing unless you make a completely unrealistic request.

Be Prepared to Sell Yourself

When offered an amount that is considerably less than you had hoped for, you might say after a slight pause, "I was hoping you would come in closer to [whatever amount you were hoping for or a little higher], based on the level of responsibility and skill required to do the job." Then you have some room to negotiate down, if necessary. If the money is there, then the negotiating begins. You can always come down with your salary requests, but you can't go up once you've stated a number. When you can't get the money you want, you can try to negotiate vacation time, tuition reimbursement, or other things that come out of a different budget.

Frequently Asked Questions

Q: *What if I'm offered a job on the spot?*

A: While this can be very flattering, it is always best to take some time to think over everything just discussed and be certain this is what you want. You could respond with, "Wow, that is tempting. I would appreciate the opportunity to sleep on it before giving you my final answer." There is nothing wrong with this, and it shows you are intelligent and logical rather than impulsive or desperate!

Q: *Is it ever OK to ask for a tour of the department or the facility?*

A: Yes, under certain circumstances. Since prospective employers are usually interviewing multiple candidates, it may not be appropriate to ask for a department or facility tour on an initial interview. It would be very time consuming for an employer to bring every job candidate around. If you are brought back for a second interview that would be an appropriate time to ask for a tour. Of course, if a tour is offered at any time, accept.

Q: *What if I'm offered a job I don't want?*

A: If that happens, tell the employer that after considering everything, you have decided this is not the right position for you so you will have to decline. Thank them for their time and interest and wish them luck in their search. If they ask for more specifics as to why, you can phrase your reasons diplomatically, such as, "This is too much of a lateral move for me," or "I realize I would prefer to do something more clinical in scope." They may say, "Is there anything we can do to change your mind?" If there is something, such as more money, let them know. If not, say so.

Q: *What if I accept a job and then, for whatever reason, change my mind before I have actually started?*

A: While you should always accept a job in good faith after due consideration, you may still find yourself in this situation at one time or another. The important thing to do is to notify the prospective employer as soon as possible, ideally by telephone. If the person who interviewed you is not available, then speak to someone in HR so that the message is conveyed immediately. It is not appropriate to send this type of message by email or to leave a voice mail message; these forms of communication are unreliable and are too informal to convey such a message. *It is never appropriate to simply not show up on your designated start date as a way of getting your message across.* Remember, you never know when you'll run into the people who interviewed or hired you at another time in another location. Your behavior—good or bad—will follow you wherever you go.

Q: *What if they ask if they can contact my current employer?*

A: If you are job searching while employed elsewhere, the likelihood is that your current employer doesn't know you're looking nor would you want them to. Simply answer this question by saying, "No. Not at this time." That is perfectly normal and understood. It will not be held against you. In this circumstance, a recruiter may request from the candidate a copy of the their last performance evaluation, which has the evaluator's and candidate's signatures. This is another good reason why it's always good to request and retain copies of your performance evaluations.

Q: *What if my former company or facility has closed, been sold, or moved? How do I explain that on a job application or reference check form?*

A: These things happen, so just be straightforward about it. If the company is closed, you can list the employer but in the address section you can state, "Closed" or, "No longer in business." If the company or facility has been sold or acquired and now operates under a new name, list the name and address used when you worked there and add in parenthesis: "(Currently known as [current name if you know it])." If a company relocated and you have lost track of them, in the address section of an application you can note: "Relocated. Current address unknown."

Q: *What if my former supervisors no longer work where I did? Whom can I use as work references?*

A: For starters, your work references do not have to still work in the place where you worked with them, so that is not a problem. However, if an employer specifically wants to speak to a past supervisor or director from a particular job and that person no longer works there, you would simply tell that to the interviewer. This scenario is fairly common since so many people change jobs so often these days. However, if you've lost track of them, you can try to find them on LI or other social media.

Q: *How much can and will a previous employer reveal about my past?*

A: Today, most employers are cautious about what they say about former employees. Some have a policy of only verifying titles and employment dates. That's not always the case with former supervisors. And remember, if you're applying for a patient care position, some states have laws regarding mandatory disclosure of certain information when requested by prospective health care employers related to clinical practice and patient care issues. We discussed how to deal with a problematic past in chapter 7.

This is one reason why it is best to be honest and upfront about these situations if they exist in your employment history. If you conceal something like this and the employer finds out about it later, you will almost definitely be disqualified from the position. However, if you disclose the situation and address it adequately, the prospective employer may be willing to hire you in spite of it, depending on the situation.

Interviewing Essentials—A Review
- Be well prepared
- Be impeccably dressed and groomed

- Arrive early and take time to ground yourself
- Smile, make eye contact, and shake hands
- Be attentive, conversational, and ask questions
- Show interest in the job, the company, and the interviewer
- Every interviewer's style is different, so go with flow
- Think in terms of what the interviewer is interested in
- Bring extra copies of your résumé and business card
- Be courteous to everyone you encounter
- Let your personality shine through
- Turn negatives into positives
- Project a positive, upbeat, can-do attitude
- Act confident even if you don't feel confident
- End the interview on a positive note
- Send a short text or email shortly after the interview (same day)
- Send a typed thank-you note via USPS within 24 hours
- Follow up with a phone call if necessary

When all is said and done, the majority of employers hire people (or don't) because of their personality. A positive, upbeat, can-do attitude is worth more to many employers than all the credentials and experience in the world.

Choosing the Right Job for You

In deciding whether or not to accept a job offer, go back to the basics discussed in chapter 3 about where to go from here. Reflect on what type of work you enjoy doing and what your ideal work environment and schedule would be like, then contemplate how well this position meets those needs and interests. Think about how your lifestyle, including your family life if applicable, will be affected. Consider your commute, amount of paid vacation and personal time, and whether or not you would have to work holidays or weekends, or do shift work. Can you telecommute? Is the schedule flexible? What type of support staff is available to help you to do your job well? What is the dress code? And so on.

When all is said and done, the work and the company should provide an opportunity for you to learn and grow professionally. The work should be something that is interesting and even exciting to you. You should get paid a fair wage for your experience, credentials, and education. The schedule and workload should support your ability to have a good quality of life that includes time for your family and friends and your own self-care.

When accepting a job, ask to get the offer, including the salary and any special benefits discussed, *in writing*. Getting it in writing not only makes the offer official, but you have some documentation in case there is a discrepancy about what was agreed upon later. It has been known to happen. Look out for your own best interests.

How to Resign from Your Current Job

Once you've accepted a job and received the offer in writing, the first thing you must do if you're currently working elsewhere is notify your current boss. Don't tell anyone, other than your immediate family, about your new job until you have told your boss. Word gets around no matter how discreet you may be, and your boss should never hear about your resignation from someone else! I have seen it happen on more than one occasion. In fact, someone who worked under me told her friend in a distant city about a new job she accepted. She was going to wait a few weeks before resigning because she wanted to collect some benefits that would accrue. Her friend just happened to know a good friend of mine and mentioned it to her, not knowing it was supposed to be a secret. I of course heard about it and confronted my staff member. She was embarrassed beyond belief and did not leave on good terms as a result.

Every employer should have a policy related to resignation protocol, including how much notice must be given, so be sure to check that policy before doing anything. When notifying your current boss about your resignation, it is ideal to tell them in person. If you can't tell your boss in person in a timely manner, then resort to the telephone. This should be followed up in writing immediately. It is always a good idea to give one copy to your boss and another to HR. This way, no one can claim they didn't know, or that you didn't give proper notice. Cover all your bases.

When writing your letter of resignation (see sample at end of chapter) and when informing your boss that you are leaving, it is best to stay professional with your words and your demeanor, regardless of the reasons that you are leaving. In other words, don't burn your professional bridges; it will never serve you well in life. Even if you don't like your job, your boss, or the company you work for, always write a professional letter of resignation. The purpose of the letter is to notify your employer that you are resigning. It is *not* the place to air your grievances. This letter will become part of your permanent record.

Some employers will conduct an exit interview with all employees before they leave. The purpose of this session is to learn more about why you're leaving and what, if anything, the employer could have done to keep you onboard. This information can be helpful to the employer for future recruitment and retention efforts. It can also help them to address internal problems if applicable. This is not a gripe session. Nor is it an opportunity to disparage someone you didn't get along with. However, if you are leaving because of unresolved problems or other issues such as short staffing or a hostile workplace, be constructive and professional in your remarks.

Here's another reason to leave on professional terms: You never know who might be sitting behind the desk 5 years from now at another company or facility when you go on an interview. Also, people know people who know other people, and your actions will have a ripple effect whether positive or negative. The choice is yours.

In chapter 9 we'll discuss some additional job-hunting and career challenges as well as advice and information for some unique and special situations in nursing, including various phases of a nurse's career.

Sample Resignation Letter
©Donna Cardillo. Reprinted with permission.

Janice Smith, RN, ADN
45 Lane Avenue
Smithville, NJ, 00090
Cell: 908-555-8686
jsmith@net.net

November 11, 20__

Mary Harris, RN
Director of Quality Management
Allenwood Hospital
311 City Street
Allenwood, NJ 22536

Dear Ms. Harris,

Per our conversation earlier today, I am resigning my position as staff nurse effective December 11, 20__. I have accepted a position as a utilization review nurse with Health International.

I have enjoyed working at Allenwood Hospital and thank you for the opportunities afforded me.

Best of luck to you. I hope our paths cross again in the future.

Sincerely,

Janice Smith, RN, ADN

Janice Smith, RN, ADN

Sample Thank-You Letter

©Donna Cardillo. Reprinted with permission.

Janice Smith, RN, ADN
45 Lane Avenue
Smithville, NJ 00090
908-555-8686
jsmith@net.net

November 11, 20__

Mary Harris, RN
Director of Quality Management
Allenwood Hospital
11 City Street
Allenwood, NJ 22536

Dear Ms. Harris,

It was a pleasure meeting and speaking with you today. I am convinced that the position of Quality Assurance Coordinator at Allenwood Hospital is the right job for me and that I can contribute substantially to the department and the facility.

My strong clinical background combined with my excellent communication skills will allow me to do the job that needs to be done. Also, I am reliable, detail oriented, and motivated to succeed.

If I can provide you with any additional information, please do not hesitate to contact me. Thank you for your time, and I look forward to speaking with you again soon.

Sincerely,

Janice Smith, RN, ADN

Janice Smith, RN, ADN

Chapter 9

Special Situations and Career Challenges

Now that we've covered general job search and career management strategies, it's time to address specific situations and challenges that may occur at one time or another over the course of a nurse's career.

Job-Hunting Challenges

So far, we addressed what to do when you go on an interview and accept a job offer. But what if your job search isn't going as well as you'd like? Maybe you're not getting any interviews, or you're getting interviews but not getting any job offers. Here are some common challenges related to job hunting along with strategies to overcome them.

Challenge 1: You're Sending Out Résumés but Not Getting Responses

This could be happening for several reasons. Here are a few possibilities along with recommended solutions:

- Your résumé and cover letter may be working against you. Look them over and ask yourself, Are they as good as they could be? Are they written in an up-to-date format that showcases your unique experiences and presents you and your background in a positive light? Review résumé writing and cover letter basics in chapters 5 and 6. Ask someone who hires or coaches nurses to look at your résumé and cover letter and give you some feedback.

• You could be using the wrong approach to job finding for the type of position you're going after or the industry you want to get into; take another tack. Network more, do informational interviewing, consider part-time or temporary work to break into the field or gain experience, and consider volunteering as a way to get your foot in the door somewhere.

Challenge 2: You're Going on Interviews but Not Getting Any Offers

Remember, there is a lot of competition out there, especially for the good jobs. Consider the following strategies to increase your chances of getting a job offer:

• Review interview basics in chapters 7 and 8. Are you doing everything you could be doing, as well as you can? Are you dressing appropriately? Are you able to answer usual questions and market yourself well? Are you able to articulate your strengths and assets? Are you following up as recommended in chapter 8? Be honest in your self-assessment and work on improving your image, your technique, and your form. Use a career coach if necessary.

• If you interviewed with someone you felt comfortable with, call them shortly after you find out you did not get the job. Tell them that you are working on perfecting your interview skills, that you respect their opinion as a professional, and that you were wondering if they could give you any suggestions on how you might improve your performance in the future. You would, of course, say this in a very friendly, nonchalant way, so the interviewer does not feel put on the spot to explain why they didn't hire you. Many people will respect this and give you some constructive feedback. Everyone I know who has ever done this tells me that while it is difficult to do, and sometimes difficult to hear, it is some of the most valuable feedback they have ever gotten. Remember, if what you are doing isn't working, then it's time to take a new approach.

Challenge 3: Never Hearing Back

After an interview, you should follow up with a thank-you note and a phone call or email if necessary, as described in chapter 8. In some cases you may need to make several attempts to contact someone from the company (the person or people who interviewed you and/or someone in human resources [HR]) to see what your status is. You can try making contact on LinkedIn (LI), too. Unfortunately, there are times that an employer just never gets back to candidates. So if, after repeated attempts at follow-up, you still haven't gotten anywhere, you may need to just move on.

If a week or two has passed after you sent in a résumé, and you haven't heard anything, it is appropriate to call to be sure your résumé was received. However, if you respond to a blind classified ad—one that does not identify the employer or provide a phone number—then you have little recourse for follow-up.

Assimilating into a New Position, Workplace, or Specialty

Whether you're thinking about changing jobs, getting ready to move into a new role, or returning to the workforce, it will be necessary for you to learn new things, meet new people, and step out of your comfort zone. In chapter 3 we discussed challenges to moving forward that included coping with fear, risk avoidance, indecision, and excuse making. Be sure to reread that section whenever you are in the midst of change in your career. That being said, the following are practical strategies to help you make a successful transition in a variety of situations.

Changing Specialties

In chapter 3 we discussed how to research various specialties and positions before making a decision to move. Once you've made that decision and have landed a job, it's important to take steps to acclimate yourself to your new specialty:

1. Immediately join and get active in a related professional association such as the Emergency Nurses Association (ENA; www.ena. org), Academy of Medical-Surgical Nurses (www.amsn.org), or the American Holistic Nurses Association (AHNA; www.ahna.org). You'll immediately start to get the association publications, and you'll be able to access members-only sections of their web sites. Some associations even provide online mentoring or chat rooms where you can tap into the wisdom of nurses experienced in any specialty. This will significantly increase your learning curve.

2. Get out to local chapter meetings of your specialty association, as well as state and national conventions and conferences. Go by yourself or ask your new coworkers who belong if you can tag along with them. You'll benefit from the education, information exchange, support, and networking at these events. Remember that while no one thinks they have "extra time" to network, networking will actually energize you and support your career in many ways.

3. Find out what books and other resources exist related to your new specialty. Do an online book and article search, check with the related professional association, and ask others who work in the

specialty for recommendations. Immerse yourself in self-directed study. Don't rely on your employer to provide all of your education and training. Become an expert on your own.

It's always scary to move in a new direction with your career, especially when you've developed some expertise in another area. While some nurses may consider changing specialties as "starting over again," that is hardly the case. Sure you'll have things to learn in your new setting, but you'll be expanding your knowledge base and experience and building on what you already know rather than starting from scratch. The knowledge from prior positions will probably have unexpected contributions to make as well. It's all in how you look at it.

Transitioning from Traditional to Nontraditional Nursing Roles

When making a transition from a traditional patient care position to something less traditional, such as case management, telephone triage, or legal nurse consulting, it is common for some nurses to feel uneasy. I've heard nurses refer to this as "changing careers" or "leaving nursing," neither of which is the case. The truth is that, as outlined in chapter 1, nurses are versatile and multi-talented. We are scientists, healers, teachers, and nurturers. There are many ways and places to make a difference—some direct and some indirect. We are vital at the bedside, but we are just as vital in every other aspect of the health care arena.

Is a nurse who works for an insurance company, who is an editor of a nursing magazine, who is a recruiter for a hospital, or who does research any less a nurse than one who delivers direct patient care? Not at all.

Actually, the more places we work, the greater impact we will have as health care experts and as patient advocates, the more we will get noticed and taken seriously, and the louder our collective voice will be. Besides, having options is a good thing. Just knowing you have options lessens your anxiety about the future.

When moving into a nontraditional role, not only will you have things to learn about your new specialty, but you may also be working in a different type of environment and be required to learn different types of skills. You may even be required to dress differently than you are accustomed to, e.g., business clothes instead of uniforms or scrubs. Because of this, many nurses when making such a transition will say, "I feel like a fish out of water." That feeling is normal and will dissipate as time goes on. Unfortunately, some nurses jump ship and return to their old jobs before giving themselves an opportunity to become comfortable in their new setting. Every new job, specialty, and work setting requires a period of adjustment. You have to set small, short-term goals for yourself and track your progress. Remind yourself that you are expanding your horizons and your experience base every day. Also, expand your view of who you are, what you do, and what you are capable of doing as a nurse.

Going from Expert to Novice

One fear particular to nurses in the process of making changes in their professional life is the fear of going from expert to novice. Many nurses have worked in a particular specialty, and in some cases, even for the same employer, for many years. They can handle everything that comes up. They know the language, the routine, and the people. They know how to answer all the questions that come up, and that's a very comfortable place to be.

You may be able to deduct all or part of your professional development expenses and fees, including travel expenses, dues, and book purchase price, so check with your tax preparer.

Then, when they consider advancing in their position, changing specialties or employers (whether by choice or not), or moving in a completely new direction like entrepreneurship or teaching, they will have a lot to learn and may feel like a novice for a time. The security of "knowing it all" is gone.

Here are a few helpful things to remember when making a change in your career:

1. Nurses have above-average intelligence. What do I base this on? The fact that you made it through a strenuous educational program, passed a rigorous state licensing exam, and worked in the complex and ever-changing world of health care.

2. Whether you realize it or not, you've constantly had to learn new things and been thrown into situations where you weren't always sure of yourself. You'll apply those same skills and abilities to any new practice setting you go after. And the way I look at it, you've already learned the hardest stuff in nursing school and in your first nursing job. Anything else is simply an expansion of what you already know and already do.

3. You only have to do something for the first time once. After you've done something even one time, you immediately start to gain experience.

4. It only takes 3–6 months to master a new skill. So when you start something new, you have to set small goals for yourself. Tell yourself, OK, in 3 months I'm going to have a grip on the situation; in 6 months I'll be working pretty independently, and in 1 year it will be as if I've always been here. Keep in mind that each day on a new job or in a new role, you become more experienced than you were the day before.

Additional Strategies

In addition to learning about your new specialty or practice area when making any career change, it is important to take steps to assimilate into your new work environment. This involves getting to know staff members, becoming part of the team, understanding the corporate culture, and learning about systems, procedures, and equipment. I write extensively about these things in my book *Your First Year as a Nurse: Making the Transition from Total Novice to Successful Professional.* Although the book was written for newly licensed nurses, sometimes it is helpful to go back to basics when making transitions. And since some of us never learned the basics to begin with, a review may provide some valuable information for being successful in your career at any phase.

To summarize, here are some key points included in *Your First Year as a Nurse*: Go out of your way to introduce yourself to staff members in all departments and on all shifts. Learn and use people's names. Greet people when you arrive to work each day and say goodbye at the end of the workday. Participate in work-related social events. Make an effort to get to know your coworkers by having lunch with different people occasionally and just by showing interest in them. Be willing to learn from all of your experienced coworkers regardless of their title or position. Treat everyone with respect and be willing to help out as needed even if something is "not your job." Don't be afraid to ask questions or ask for help when you need it.

Going into Advanced Practice

There are more and more nurses going into advanced practice (e.g., becoming nurse practitioners, clinical nurse specialists, certified nurse midwives, certified registered nurse anesthetists) these days for a variety of reasons. Of those who complete the requirements, many are very successful, yet some never manage to get a foothold in their new role. This has less to do with the job market since advanced practice nurses (APNs) are working in an increasing number of roles and settings. It has more to do with APNs' ability to market and promote themselves—something many nurses find difficult to do.

Once you've elevated your degree, your certifications, and your level of practice, you also have to elevate your image, your expectations, your social skills, and your career management expertise. Also, you need to develop an expanded view of your new role in health care. Many APNs are still staff nurses at heart and haven't fully taken ownership of their new level of practice. They aren't able to see themselves in a new role. This can become a bigger obstacle than you might imagine.

I often hear new APNs say, "I have no experience," or, "I'm just starting out." On the contrary, you already have many years of nursing experience

When I was a kid, I took swimming lessons at a local high school. After mastering some basics strokes, it was time to jump off the diving board into the deep end of the pool in order to advance to the next level. I had only swum in 3-foot-deep water so far and was scared to death to jump into water over my head—so much so that I considered dropping out of swimming.

And yet, as scared as I was, my desire to advance in the swimming program was strong. So I devised a plan such as it was—to get me through. When the big day came, I decided I would walk to the edge of the board quickly, close my eyes, hold my nose, jump in, and pray that I wouldn't drown. It was one of the hardest and scariest things I ever did in my life. By some miracle (or so I felt it to be), I survived the impact, came to the surface, and swam to the edge of the pool. Frightening as it was, the whole thing wasn't nearly as bad as I had anticipated.

Isn't that always the way? Our fears are usually greater than the reality of a situation. I now had some "experience" under my belt. My second jump was a little easier and the third jump easier still because I knew what to expect and was a little better prepared. Before I knew it, the diving board became fun.

This was a great lesson—one that I still carry with me. To this day, whenever I have something scary to do for the first time, in my mind I walk quickly to the edge of the board, close my eyes, hold my nose, jump in, and pray. Whatever I have to face in life, using this mental technique, I always manage to "survive the impact, come to the surface, and swim to the side of the pool." Things always get easier after that.

(unless you are an APN entry to practice). You are simply expanding your experience and practice, *not* starting from scratch; you are taking your practice to the next level, *not* starting from square one. This is an important distinction to make.

Consider the following strategies to make the most of your advanced practice status:

1. **Polish your professional image.** Have business cards made with your new credentials, dress well, and master assertive body language. Pay attention to the social graces, including using a full firm handshake in workplace or business and social settings. Remember, you can act confident even if you don't feel confident. You have to inspire confidence in others.

2. **Build a support system of peers.** Create a network of APNs for support, information exchange, and networking. One way to do this is to join and get active in your specialty association as well as a related advanced practice association. This means getting out to occasional meetings, conferences, conventions, and special programs. It may also mean getting on committees, running for office in the association, or working on special projects. It is critical to stay connected to your peers at this level of practice. Look for role models and mentors for inspiration, information, encouragement, and support.

3. **Develop a new job-finding strategy.** Don't rely on traditional methods to find jobs such as classified ads. Most advanced practice positions are filled through networking or word of mouth. That means you have to get on the phone with all of your professional colleagues—physicians, nurses, administrators, and anyone else you know in the industry. Let them know of your new credentials and tell them what you're looking for. Ask for advice, when appropriate, and for referrals.

   Get in the habit of introducing yourself with your new credentials to others in workplace and social situations. You never know whom you'll meet where. As mentioned throughout this book, the power of networking is far reaching. Besides, when you meet people and tell them you're an APN, that's a great opportunity for them to ask you questions about your role to promote understanding and acceptance of APNs.

4. **Consider alternate practice settings.** Look into opportunities in community health centers, clinics, collaborative practice with other physicians and APNs, and even self-employment. While traditional hospital employment may be what you are accustomed to, it's time to broaden your horizons and consider all of your options. Not only will this expand your opportunities, it may lead to more money, flexibility, and autonomy.

Do some informational interviewing with seasoned APNs to learn from their experience. Attend seminars and read books on self-employment, contract negotiation, and related professional issues. In other words, learn about the "business" of being an APN:

1. **Learn to sell yourself.** Rather than looking for an "opening" to fill, you may have to sell your new credentials to an employer or organization and actually create your own position and job description. You might also have to sell your role when an employer is looking for another type of professional. I know more than one APN who applied for a position when the employer was looking for a physician assistant. In each case the APN was able to convince the employer that an APN added more value to the position and would be a better choice. Don't assume that all employers understand your role in health care and will automatically create positions for you.

   Once you land a job, enter into a collaborative practice, or start a business, continue to promote your role. Do this by creating brochures or fact sheets about what APNs do. Talk to colleagues and coworkers about your role and how they can best use your specialized knowledge and expertise. Explain to patients, in language they can understand, what it means to be an APN and what your role is—how you will be working with them and how you can help them. Just because you exist and have a spiffy new credential and title, it does not mean that those around you will automatically know what to do with you or understand your unique role. Self-promotion is self-preservation for the individual and the practice.

2. **Work on your communication skills.** Read books and take courses in effective oral and written communication. This includes conversational communication, writing for business (letters, memos, proposals), public speaking, and writing for publication. As an APN you will be communicating with a broader range of people on a broader range of topics. It is imperative that you develop excellent communication skills on every level.

   Also, it is imperative that you develop your professional practice and expand your sphere of influence through professional speaking and writing. Public speaking and writing for publication not only boost your credibility and visibility, they also help position you as an expert as well as showcase the role and expertise of all APNs. And, of course, they allow you to reach more people with your specialized knowledge and therefore have a greater impact. Don't restrict your writing and speaking to other nurses; target consumer audiences, physician groups, and other health care professionals as well.

Moving into Management

If you aspire to get into a management position, take these positive steps:

1. **Work on your education.** An advanced degree will make you well rounded; more knowledgeable about systems, theory, and practice; and more marketable. It will also increase your confidence.

2. **Join a related management association.** The American Organization of Nurse Executives (AONE; www.aone.org) is open to all nurses regardless of their role or level of experience. Here you'll find role models, mentors, support, and education. Get active in your local chapter. The National Association of Directors of Nursing Administration in Long Term Care (NADONA; www.nadona.org) is open to all nurses who work in long-term care. The American College of Healthcare Executives (ACHE; www.ache.org) requires a minimum of a bachelor's degree and a commitment to the profession of health care management for membership.

3. **Seek out related assignments at work.** Look for those that will help you build related skills, such as working on the budget, schedule, policies, and procedures. Get active on committees and special projects. All of these things will propel you forward in your career, make you more visible in your workplace, and build your confidence as well as your skill set.

4. **Let your supervisor, manager, or director know about your aspirations.** A good manager will support you in your goals by providing related learning experiences and considering or recommending you for positions when they come up.

Once you have a management position, even a supervisor's role:

1. **Immerse yourself in self-directed study.** Read and take courses related to the management of people in general as well as nursing and health care management. Just because you have the title or the responsibility doesn't mean you automatically become an effective leader. Management is not a skill you learn by experience alone. And you cannot rely exclusively on your employer to provide all of the support and education you need to be successful in your new role.

2. **Seek role models and mentors.** Look for individuals both at work and through your professional associations to model yourself after and for support and advice. If you haven't already joined AONE, NADONA, or ACHE, what are you waiting for? You should also belong to your state association of ANA and specialty association. Remember: *No one succeeds alone.* Besides, this is the best way to stay on the cutting edge with knowledge and information about your specialty, about trends in nursing and health care, and about effective management techniques and tools.

3. **Work on professional development skill-building.** In addition to continuously developing your clinical and managerial skills, work on your communication skills, professional image, conflict management, and negotiation skills. All of these are necessary to be an effective leader. You set the tone for your department. You set the example. You must model the behavior you want to see in your staff. It is a big responsibility; take it seriously.

Phases of a Nurse's Career

There are various stages in nurses' careers, where our needs, our interests, and our experiences are different. Here are some tips to help you successfully navigate through the most common phases.

Student Nurse

Nursing is the toughest job you'll ever love. In addition to your formal education and training while a student nurse, there are many additional things that you can do to prepare for your future career and give yourself a competitive edge. Here are several:

Make the most of your classes and clinical time. Show up and participate. Do your own research and reading, ask questions, and ask for help when you need it. This is a special time to learn from experienced nurses—your instructors—and get all the nurturing and guidance you can.

Join and get active in the National Student Nurses' Association (NSNA; www.nsna.org). Joining NSNA has many tangible benefits. For starters, you will receive publications targeted to student nurses with pertinent articles, insights, book reviews, and more. You'll stay abreast of upcoming conventions and special programs. Many schools will allow students time off to attend these conventions. Also, membership looks good on your résumé and will make you more marketable. There are many leadership opportunities within the association that you may wish to take advantage of. I know of one hospital system that markets specifically to NSNA members because they are viewed by some as the cream of the crop.

Consider part-time work in health care. The more clinical experience and exposure that you get during your student years, the more comfortable and confident you will feel upon graduation. You will also significantly increase your learning curve. So if your schedule allows it and your school permits it, look for work as a nurse's aide, patient care technician, emergency room technician, emergency medical technician (EMT), and so on. Some of these positions require specific training and certification courses, but others do not.

Some health care facilities offer student externships, which are paying jobs often offered in the summer months, specifically for student nurses. These programs have more structure and support and allow you to work with experienced nurses in various specialties. You will often have an opportunity to do even more during an externship than you might in a regular job as an aide or technician.

It is ideal to seek work, including externships, in a facility where you may wish to work after graduation. This will allow you to become familiar with the physical plant as well as many of the people and procedures. And while this does not guarantee that the facility will hire you afterward, it certainly can't hurt, especially if you have made a good impression.

Consider volunteering. Volunteering is also an excellent way to gain experience, make valuable contacts, and find ongoing support for your budding nursing career from experienced, competent, and enthusiastic nursing professionals. Consider offering to help out at health fairs provided by your local department of health or by a local health care organization.

Contact organizations such as the American Red Cross, American Heart Association, or other social service agencies of interest to you about volunteer opportunities. Look into opportunities in hospice care, adult day care, long-term care, and so forth.

Get out and network. Networking is a great way to make valuable contacts, learn about student and graduate nurse opportunities, and to find mentors and role models. Whenever possible, attend nursing conventions, conferences, career fairs, and so on. Fortunately, most schools of nursing encourage and support these activities; take advantage of them. Be sure to bring business cards and résumés along!

Join a specialty association. If you happen to have a special interest in obstetrics, perioperative, emergency, or other kinds of nursing, join the related specialty association as a student member. Most nursing associations have such a membership category and the dues are nominal. This will provide an opportunity to learn more about the specialty, gain access to experienced members of the specialty, and give access to member's-only areas of the web site if applicable. It will increase your learning curve and give you a competitive edge if you decide to enter that specialty upon graduation.

New Graduate

Between graduation and licensing, there is that unique time of relief, anticipation, dread, fear, and celebration. It is a time of transition between student and licensed nurse. There are many things you can do during this time to facilitate a smooth transition.

Celebrate! Once you've graduated, take time to revel in your accomplishment and do something special to celebrate. Take some time off, if possible, to de-stress and bask in the glow of your accomplishment. Reward yourself in a constructive way for all of your hard work with a vacation, spa day, favorite activity, or time with friends and family. Just don't let that time off delay your preparation for the NCLEX (the National Council Licensure Examination).

Prepare for your licensing exam. To prepare for taking your licensing exam, it is helpful to use some review books to acquaint yourself with the types of questions that will be asked. You can find NCLEX review books in your school library, the public library, bookstores, and online. You can even find some free resources on the Internet. Most new graduates benefit from a more intensive review offered by education companies by way of live or online classes (many schools offer this to their graduates). There are also private tutors available who specialize in working with new grads to achieve NCLEX success. Review as necessary but don't overstudy. This is not an exam you can cram for. At this point you either know the material, or you don't.

In addition to material review, be sure to study strategies for successful test taking. Going through sample test questions helps familiarize you with the process and get into the exam groove. It's important to remember that licensing exams test basic knowledge; they are not designed to trick

A certain percentage of new graduates don't pass NCLEX the first time. If it happens to you, don't despair. It's happened to more people than you might imagine. Once you get your license, no one will know how many times you took the test before passing. Go through the above steps again, this time with even greater resolve. Be sure to think positively. Picture yourself as a licensed nurse looking back on this time in your early career.

or deceive. Just before the test, take time to de-stress and relax so you'll be well rested and focused. Use positive visualization—imagine yourself acing the test and passing with flying colors.

Note: Research shows that the sooner you take NCLEX after graduation, the better your chances of passing, so don't delay.

Newly Licensed Nurse
Get Connected

If you want a successful career in nursing, you must immerse yourself in the community of nursing. Staying isolated will lead to unhappiness and a feeling of being overwhelmed, and will pave the road to burnout. Once you are a licensed nurse, join and get active in your state nurses association. Once you've secured your first job, also join a related specialty association if you're not already a member, such as the American Association of Critical-Care Nurses (AACN; www.aacn.org). Tap into the wonderful support and resources that already exist in nursing rather than trying to go it alone. As a reminder, some associations offer online and other forms of mentoring to new graduates. Use everything that is available to you!

Choosing Your First Job

In choosing your first job, look for a facility that offers a long and comprehensive new nurse orientation program complete with preceptor, ideally 6 months in length or longer. Some facilities also offer mentors in addition to preceptors. Mentors are usually nurses who you do not work with on a daily basis but who will meet with you to discuss how things are going and advise and support you in various ways.

If you have an interest in working in a particular specialty such as trauma, intensive care, or psych, find out if that specialty is available to a newly licensed nurse at that facility and what type of specialty internship or specialized training is provided. I'm often asked, "Is it necessary to do 2 years of medical-surgical nursing before going into a specialty?" While medical-surgical (also called med-surg) is a good place for some nurses to start, it is not right for every nurse. There is no one right path for all nurses to follow. Every nurse must follow their heart and carve out their own career path.

If you're not sure what you want to do, consider starting out on a med-surg or telemetry floor where you'll be exposed to many different types of patients and procedures. If you're offered a position in a particular specialty simply because an opening exits in that department, research the specialty and the unit before making a commitment. Sometimes fate steps in and makes up your mind for you by presenting an opportunity you might not have otherwise considered.

Keep in mind that while salary is important to everyone, it should not be a primary factor in choosing your first job. What is most important is that you find a position in a facility that will best support your role as a new graduate nurse and nurture your growth and development. This is a pivotal time in your career. Your first job will help lay the foundation for the rest of your career.

Once Working

Keep in mind that nursing school was phase one of your education. Your first job as a licensed nurse is phase two. You still have much to learn and are not expected to know everything or do everything. Seasoned nurses will tell you that it takes a full year before you start to feel some level of confidence. It will take another year before you begin to develop some level of competency. Don't be discouraged. You'll be moving forward the entire time and gaining confidence and experience. And believe me, the destination is worth the journey. Here are a few tips to help you along the way:

- **Align yourself with friendly, competent nurses.** They are all over if you only look for them. Contrary to what you may have heard, the vast majority of nurses are supportive, professional, and happy to help and guide you.

- **Be proactive with your training.** Don't wait for someone to show you how to do something. Ask to observe, assist, or perform a procedure with an experienced nurse when the opportunity arises. Seek opportunities to learn.

- **Watch, listen, and learn.** Read policy and procedure manuals and utilize other resources on your unit. Ask questions when you need to. Learn from your experienced coworkers regardless of their title or position. An experienced tech, aide, or unit clerk has a lot of knowledge to share and can teach you tricks of the trade.

- **Offer to help others.** Even though you are inexperienced, you can help turn or transport a patient, get supplies if needed, make a bed, and so on. When you extend yourself to others, they will reciprocate.

- **Respect everyone you work with.** Always say thank you when someone helps you. Everyone is on the same team and each person plays a vital role.

- **Work on staying positive and focused.** It's easy to get down when you feel challenged and overwhelmed. Keep a journal, use motivational audio recordings and books, and keep a record of your progress and accomplishments. Record positive things that patients, staff, and family members say to you and make note how you are making a difference.

- **Advocate for yourself.** If you don't get along with your preceptor, speak to your manager or the nurse responsible for your orientation. If you're not getting enough exposure to different types of procedures or cases, ask for additional opportunities.

- **Immerse yourself in the community of nursing.** Join and get active in your state association of ANA and specialty association. Create alliances, build support, and get connected. Staying isolated serves no useful purpose.

The Second-Career New Nurse

Many nurses are coming to the profession later in life, possibly as a second, third, or fourth career. It could be a homemaker in her 50s or 60s who never had a career outside of the home and always wanted to be nurse but just never had the chance. It could be a 40-year-old woman with an MBA and 15 years of management experience in the business world who would like to do something where she feels she is making a positive difference in people's lives. It could be a 60-year-old or older man who owned a business for most of his life and is looking for something meaningful to do in his "retirement." It could also be a 30-something-year-old man who has been working in the computer industry, now looking for a career where he can make a real contribution while making a good salary and benefits with opportunities for advancement.

The truth is that new nurses have diverse backgrounds these days, and not every employer has adapted well to that diversity. Don't be surprised if some of your managers don't seem to know how to react to you because you have more management experience than they do, or if people assume you're experienced or that you're ready to retire because of your age. Take it all with a grain of salt and focus on the task at hand—honing your nursing knowledge and skills.

If you come from a business or corporate background, you will likely find the health care culture to be very different in a variety of ways, so be prepared. Although every place of employment is different, you may experience remnants of the old patriarchal days of health care when physicians ruled. You may find some new nurse training programs to be geared toward the young, inexperienced learner. You may also encounter some nurses from the "old school" who believe that nurses should stay separate and not participate in facility-wide events, committees, or boards.

When the time feels right, which will be after you've gained some nursing experience and have assimilated well into your new unit, offer to work on some projects or develop some educational programs where you can utilize skills, specialized knowledge, and talents that you acquired outside of nursing. Second-career nurses bring a broad range of unique skills, experiences, and credentials to nursing that have the potential to enrich and expand the profession in many ways.

Older Nurses

Let's face it, most of us are living and working longer. Retirement is being redefined and some have suggested that the word may be phased out of our vocabulary. That doesn't mean we can't kick back and slow down a bit in our older years—if we choose to do so. The truth is that many of us want to remain in the workforce in some capacity. Fortunately, the industry we work in recognizes and values that experience and maturity and is taking steps to accommodate us as we age.

Strategies for Older Nurses in the Workforce

That being said, some older nurses feel a bit insecure about their age and are uncertain about their marketability at this stage in life. And while age-related prejudice does exist in our society, it's important to stay up to date and relevant at every age. Here are some tips to keep you connected, confident, marketable, and competitive.

Be confident in your experience. You've accumulated a great body of life and work experience that younger people don't have. Share it, but stay open to new ideas. In other words, be willing to be both teacher and student.

Develop a contemporary look. All of us need to periodically update our hairstyle, clothing, and accessories. Styles change. Appearance matters. If your look is outdated, people can't help wondering if your knowledge and skills are outdated too.

Work at getting and staying fit. This will boost your confidence, make you look and feel better, and improve your brainpower and stamina. Many fitness clubs and programs cater to those over age 55.

Stay actively engaged in learning. Some people become intimidated by new ways of doing things as they get older. But it's the best way to stay engaged in life. Learning keeps you young, makes you feel alive, and keeps you current with knowledge, information, and skills. There is even evidence that we lose fewer brain cells due to aging if we stay actively engaged in learning new things. It's never too late to go back to school for a higher degree or even just to take some courses. Remember, education is a gift you give yourself.

Get current with technology, including social media. We often fear what we don't understand. But by taking steps to get up to date with technology of all types, we make our professional and personal lives easier, stay more connected, and remain relevant. I've suggested many ways earlier in this book to get up to speed, such as with LI.

Let go of the way things used to be. Clinging to the past is a sure way to become inconsequential. Health care and nursing, not to mention the world at large, continue to change and evolve. When you resist change, you are resisting life, happiness, and success. Keep an open mind and transform along with your surroundings.

Stay upbeat, friendly, and easygoing. Maintain a sense of fun and colleagueship in your workplace. Don't keep to yourself or only associate with those in your own age bracket. Express interest in or learn something about popular culture (e.g., movies, musicians, fashion, trends) from your kids, grandkids, or younger coworkers.

Consider alternate work settings. There are many work settings and opportunities that offer less physically demanding work and a more regular schedule if that is what you are looking for. Consider the outpatient setting and community health, such as school nursing, public health, clinics, blood banks, adult day care, and so on. There are also many nontraditional opportunities with insurance companies, private review companies, government and public agencies, and traditional health care facilities in positions such as case manager, telephone advice line nurse, disease manager, and patient advocate.

There are also some low-key positions for nurses to work in assisted living and rehabilitation facilities where you only give out medication to ambulatory or semi-ambulatory patients and do not need to provide any physical care or do any lifting.

Retiring

Retirement is a big life change. Even though some people look forward to this time of "leisure" in their lives, they often don't know what to do with themselves once they get there. Others initially enjoy traveling, spending time with family and friends, and engaging in leisure pursuits. But after a while, they long to be doing something more meaningful and constructive with their time. Some also want to continue to contribute to their community in some way.

For nurses who do wish to retire—whether on a temporary, permanent, or part-time (semiretirement) basis—there are several things you can do to stay connected to your profession. After all, nursing is not something you just turn off when you are no longer working. Many nurses experience a sense of loss or sadness when they retire and feel disconnected. But you don't have to keep working to stay connected to nursing or to contribute to your community.

It's important to stay mentally and physically active and engaged during retirement. It's fine to spend time with your grandkids, but you have to maintain your own interests, activities, leisure pursuits, and life. Here are some strategies to make the most of your retirement.

Stay connected through nursing professional associations. Even if you never belonged to anything before, join now. Consider joining your state association of ANA and/or a specialty association that you can relate to. Most associations have reduced dues for retired members. Some even have retired nurse coalitions. If yours doesn't, start one. This is a great way to stay connected and informed, maintain a sense of colleagueship, and get involved in projects when and if you feel like it.

Look into part-time work. If you want to keep working, even occasionally, contact your city and county board of health and make yourself available (on a paid or volunteer basis) to give flu shots and vaccinations or work at health fairs and public screening clinics. Contact your local board of education to do substitute school nursing or to accompany medically needy children to school in districts that offer this service. You'll find education, counseling, and other client service positions available through social service agencies such as the American Red Cross, American Heart Association, Planned Parenthood, and so on. You can also sign on with a nursing agency to be available on an occasional basis for many of the above things. This way you can stay loose with your commitments and work when and if you want to.

Consider volunteering. If you aren't necessarily interested in drawing a salary, consider volunteering in a health care setting. Many of the above settings offer volunteer opportunities. Also, schools and residences for the developmentally disabled look for "surrogate" grandparents to come in and spend time with the kids. There are opportunities everywhere.

Enjoy! Whether you continue to work part-time, volunteer, or neither, this is the perfect time in your life to engage in artistic activities, develop a new hobby, or further your education. Some people work to fill a void in their life because that's all they've ever known. Yet there are so many other things to learn—about yourself and the world around you. Grandma Moses didn't start painting until she was in her 70s!

Special Situations
Returning to the Workforce

If you've been away from the nursing workforce for some years for whatever reason, there are a number of things that you can and should do to facilitate a smooth transition back. It can be unnerving to return to work. Most people feel unsure of themselves and wonder if anyone will hire them. It is common to be uncertain about how to get started or where to look to get reconnected to your profession and to get up to date on trends, skills, and information. Here are steps to facilitate the process and build confidence:

1. **Join and get active in ANA at the state and national level.** If you've been out of the workforce, this is a great way to get reconnected to your profession—even if you've never belonged before. It's also a great way to get current on what's happening in your profession.

2. **Start volunteering.** Since jumping right into a paid nursing position can be a bit unnerving, in addition to taking some time to find the right position, volunteering is a great way to ease your way back in. Volunteering will help you build confidence, make valuable connections, hone old skills, and learn new ones. It will also give you recent relevant experience to put on your résumé and discuss in an interview. Besides all that, volunteering often leads to paid employment. So look for volunteer opportunities in settings where you'd ideally like to work or in a setting that feels comfortable. Consider any health care facility, social service agency, clinic, public health agency, or organization.

3. **Get out to career fairs and facility open houses.** These events, advertised in local newspapers and nursing publications and web sites, are great venues to test the waters and to see what is available. Attending these events is also a perfect way to brush up on your self-marketing and networking skills, which get rusty with disuse.

Returning to Bedside Nursing

If you are an experienced nurse who wishes to return to direct patient care in an acute (hospital), subacute, or long-term care setting after an extended absence (more than a few years), then a refresher course is probably in order. An "absence" here could mean that you've been out of the workforce or that you've worked in a different type of specialty—such as case management, administration, or education—where you did not deliver traditional hands-on care.

Since every employer is different, before enrolling in any courses, make some preliminary phone calls to the nurse recruiter in area health care facilities. Find out if you are eligible for hire at this point, or if you would need to take a refresher course. Inquire as to whether each facility has a reentry program for experienced nurses returning to the bedside.

If you do wish (or need) to take a refresher course, look for one that offers a comprehensive mix of classroom and clinical time, complete with a preceptor. Refresher courses are offered by health care facilities, educational institutions, and private companies. They run anywhere from 3 to 6 months in length and generally cost $1,000 and up. Contact your state association of ANA, state board of nursing, and state hospital association to locate courses in your area. You can also do an Internet search for "RN [or LPN] refresher courses in [your state]."

If you are returning to the workforce but do not wish to return to bedside nursing, you likely will not need to take a refresher course unless you wish to, or if it is required by your state board of nursing to reactivate your license.

Nurses with Disabilities

Whether you come into nursing with a disability or develop one along the way, you have plenty of options. As I've said repeatedly, there is something for everyone in this profession. Depending on your needs, interests, and experiences, there are opportunities to work from home, in office settings, in latex-free environments, and in inpatient care settings that are less physically demanding than many traditional hospital positions. There are also adaptive devices available for those with hearing, visual, and other needs. There is no obstacle that can't be overcome with persistence and determination.

Although the Americans with Disabilities Act (ADA) prohibits a prospective employer from discriminating against someone because of a disability, it doesn't prevent someone from not hiring you without revealing their reasons. So you may need to be creative, flexible, and persistent with your approach to job finding.

You are not obligated to mention any medical condition or disability on an interview unless you would need special accommodation on the job. However, if your disability is obvious—perhaps you walk with a cane, use a wheelchair, wear dark glasses, have a tremor, or similar—you might consider saying something in passing to alleviate any concerns the employer might have about liability issues or your ability to do a job. For example, if you walk with a cane, you might nonchalantly say during the interview, "By the way, although I do use a cane to walk, I have no limitations on how long I can be on my feet—just in case you were wondering." Say this with a smile on your face to reassure the employer.

When networking and going on job interviews, focus on your experience, credentials, and skill set. Downplay any limitations or disabilities. As mentioned, if you will need special accommodation on the job, you will need to mention that at some point, but don't bring it up in the beginning. Give any prospective employer an opportunity to get to know you and to be sold on you and your background. Remember that when all is said and done, employers look for someone with a positive, upbeat, can-do personality. So wow them with your charm, excellent communication skills, enthusiasm, and professionalism.

Overcoming a Difficult Past

Many nurses have unique challenges to overcome from their past such as substance abuse, serious illness, or departure from a previous job under less than ideal circumstances. Although challenging, you can work through any of these situations with a little patience, persistence, and determination. Here are some tips to help you get your career back on track.

Work on Getting Positive and Motivated

A problematic past is likely to make you feel insecure, scared, nervous, and possibly even depressed. This can show through in your facial expressions, body language, and demeanor. I've seen it many times: someone who doesn't smile, makes limited eye contact, appears on the verge of tears, and looks generally scared and nervous. Any probing question about work history sends them into a panic.

While it is understandable that you will be uneasy and uncertain while job hunting and interviewing in this situation, it is important that you focus on your good experience, credentials, and education. Focus on your great skills and abilities and the contributions you can make. Listen to or read motivational material. Sometimes we have to hear these things from other people. Review the section on challenges to moving forward in chapter 3 and use the recommendations there.

Be Ready for Tough Questions

It is inevitable that a prospective employer will ask about your work history, especially if there are gaps or if your employment history is erratic. Be prepared with answers to questions you will likely be asked. In chapter 7, I discussed how to address interview questions related to why you left your last job when there was a problem.

In chapter 8, I discussed how to address related issues on your résumé and cover letter.

Start out Volunteering

When you have a problematic background, volunteering is an excellent way to ease your way back into the job market. It will give your day or week purpose and structure so that you don't dwell on your troubles. Too much time on your hands can play havoc with your psyche and lead to more depression and self-doubt. I discussed the benefits of volunteering earlier in this chapter in the section on returning to the workforce.

Do More Networking

As already mentioned, networking is a great way to find a job, especially when you have obstacles to overcome. That means that you need to get yourself out among "the living." Get yourself a business suit or great business outfit and start attending career fairs, conventions, and association meetings. Let colleagues and friends know that you are looking for work and ask for help. It is always easier to get a job when you have someone make a recommendation, referral, or introduction for you.

Seek Job Assistance

Most state associations of ANA have peer assistance programs for nurses in recovery from substance abuse. Contact your local association whether you are a member or not. Contact local community colleges about career counseling and seek the services of a career coach, preferably one who is a nurse. Don't try to go it alone. Use every resource that is available to you.

Give Yourself a Competitive Edge

Join and get active in some professional associations. This shows you are an involved and informed member of your profession. Besides, this is one of the best ways to stay current with knowledge and trends. Enroll in some college courses and utilize online and live continuing education courses.

Additional Questions

Q: *What do I do if I get laid off from my job?*

A: Getting laid off can be devastating. But it can also be the universe's way of telling you it's time to move on. Grieve your loss and take time to de-stress and unwind before launching a full-scale job search. A forced lapse in work is the perfect time to recharge your batteries and regroup before moving forward. Consider doing temp or agency work while you look for more regular employment.

Develop a budget and see how long you can manage by living on your savings. Think of ways you can cut back on your expenditures if necessary. You'd be amazed at how little you can live on when necessary.

It is not wise to let your health care insurance coverage lapse, especially if you or a covered family member has a preexisting condition. If your employer provided you with health care benefits, then you and your covered dependents may be eligible under the Consolidated Omnibus Budget Reconciliation Act (COBRA) for temporary continuation of health care coverage at group rates. Under COBRA, you are responsible for paying the entire cost of the premium. Your employer should be able to provide you with more information about the rules and regulations that govern COBRA, or you can contact the US Department of Labor at (866) 444-3272.

You may even be eligible for unemployment insurance, depending on the circumstances of your separation. Don't be ashamed or embarrassed to use any benefits you have coming to you.

Immediately activate your network of friends, associates, and colleagues. Get on the phone and out to networking events and let everyone know you're in the job market. Be sure to save your receipts, too, since your job-hunting expenses may be tax deductible in this situation.

Q: *I was fired from my job but believe the firing was unjust. What recourse do I have?*

A: If you believe you were treated unfairly on a job and wrongly terminated, you have several courses of action that may be appropriate. Check your employer's policy on filing grievances. Take that tack if appropriate.

You can also check with your state department of labor, which will have a web site. Representatives are available to offer advice and information on work-related issues.

Consider consulting a nurse attorney or any qualified attorney who specializes in employment law. You can find a nurse attorney through The American Association of Nurse Attorneys (www.taana.org) or from a referral through your state association of ANA (go to www.nursingworld. org and click on "Find Your State").

Q: *I've considered working for myself either as an entrepreneur, consultant, or independent contractor. How do I get started?*

A: There are many great opportunities for self-employment for nurses, and we make great business owners. Start by attending a related seminar and/ or by taking business courses through a local community college.

You'll also find some great books in the public library about business ownership, consulting, and related topics. For additional information and support, contact the US Small Business Administration (SBA; www. sba.gov) and the National Nurses in Business Association (NNBA; www. nnbanow.com).

Chapter 10

The Finishing Touches

Stop for a moment and reflect on where you are in your career and think about what you'd like to accomplish in the future. Perhaps you've been contemplating going back to school, getting certified in your specialty, or running for office in your professional association. You may even be thinking about doing more writing or speaking or transitioning into a management position. Thoughts, ideas, and dreams are great, but they don't create action—and action is what gets things done. There's no better way to create positive action in your life than setting goals.

Goals are your life's game plan. They state how you'll live, where you'll go, and how you will get there. They give you a purpose to work toward. They must be specific, exact things you want to accomplish. Everyone needs to have long- and short-term goals. A long-term goal is something you want to accomplish in the next 5 years; a short-term goal is something you want to accomplish in the next year or sooner. For example, your long-term goal is to graduate from college. The short-term goals are to research the schools offering the degree you want and to submit an application to the college of your choice.

Goals must be written down or they become daydreams. You need to look at them often. A goal must be specific, challenging, objective, measurable, and have a timeframe.

Here are some long- and short-term goals:

- Get an article published in a nursing journal within the next year
- Submit a proposal to speak (or present a poster) at a nursing conference in the next 6 months
- Obtain clinical certification within the next 3 years
- Become a part-time CPR instructor in 1 year
- Complete my MSN within 5 years
- Advance into a management position within 3 years

Write down your goals, perhaps on 3 × 5 index cards, each with an accompanying target date. Keep them where you will look at them often (e.g., your refrigerator, bathroom mirror, car dashboard). This will keep you focused and on track. Research has shown that if you don't write down your goals, you're much less likely to act on them and more inclined to forget them. It serves as a visible reminder to get moving. When you reach a goal, cross it off, and set a new one. Stretch yourself; have purpose. That's what keeps life interesting.

To start you off, here are seven items for your 3 × 5 cards.

Learn High-Tech Etiquette

Today we can reach almost anyone at any time. We have become "communication junkies," addicted to our cell phones, email, and social media (SM) messaging. Many of us suffer withdrawal when we're away from them even for a short time. And stories of unprofessional use of electronic communication are abundant. The rules, written and unwritten, for effective appropriate communication, have been evolving. But the basics remain the same.

Voice Mail

Be prepared to speak to a voice mail system whenever making a call. Know what you want to say so your message will be brief and concise. Don't ramble or speak rapidly. Enunciate clearly, giving your full name and phone number, including area code even if the other person already has it. This saves that person the time of looking it up when returning your call (don't assume everyone has caller ID). Repeat your phone number a second time slowly so the person doesn't have to keep replaying your message to get the number. It's also a good idea to mention when it would be a good time to reach you, to minimize telephone tag.

When you are returning a stranger's call, jog the other person's memory by stating what their phone call was about (if you know). That person may have called a number of other people and might not immediately remember why they called you. For example, you might say, "This is Jason Sparks returning your phone call. You left me a message inquiring about guidelines for continuing education credits."

Cell Phones

Cell phones are a vital part of our world. But misuse is rampant, especially in professional circles. So here are some simple common sense rules to follow:

- When using your cell phone in public places, avoid close proximity to other people whenever possible.
- Turn off your phone or set it to vibrate while in seminars, lectures, meetings, patient care areas, or any professional setting. Although even a vibrating phone can cause a distraction, as it is often audible to others in the immediate area.
- Never take calls during an interview (yes, this happens!), performance appraisal, or negotiation. Unless you're waiting for a kidney for transplant or the birth of a child, things can wait until you pick up your voice mail messages. Set limits.

Email

Email is still the primary means of communication for many people. Yet it is not appropriate in all circumstances and does not replace many traditional forms of communication.

For example, a formal interview thank-you note, as mentioned in chapter 8, should still be sent via the US Postal Service in most cases. You should never resign from a job, discuss a sensitive subject, or respond in an angry way through email. And since you don't have the benefit of nonverbal communication cues when using email, choose your words carefully before hitting the send button.

As a reminder, here are some email basics:

- Be formal. Write a work-related email as if you were writing a letter or memo. Use proper grammar, punctuation, spelling, and salutations. Proofread the note before sending and don't rely exclusively on spell-check. Don't use abbreviations common in SM speech, such as the letter U to replace the word "you."

- Include the sender's message. With all the email correspondence sent today, it's impossible to recall what you said to whom. So make sure you include the sender's message when you reply to an email. I've received email responses that said, "Yes. That's great." I had no idea what the person was responding to, so I had to go into my "sent" folder and search for my last email to them, if I even saved it. It's time-consuming and annoying.

- Consider skipping attachments. Because of all the computer viruses circulating today, don't send an attachment unless it's something important and to someone whom you've told to expect it. Otherwise, you run the risk of having your message deleted without being read. And larger attachments run the risk of not going through at all.

- Use a clear subject line. Giving receivers an idea about the content of your email ensures that they'll know if they need to read your email immediately. Avoid generic subject phrases like, "Hi." If the subject changes after several messages, change the subject line, too.

- Email is not always as reliable as we assume, so ask for confirmation of receipt of important and time-sensitive emails. Follow up with a text message or phone call if you don't get a timely response on something important.

- When using email for professional purposes, it makes sense to create a "signature" that includes your full name, title and company (if appropriate), preferred email address, phone number, plus website (if applicable) and your SM links. This makes it easy for others to stay in touch, enter you into their contacts database, and know exactly with whom they are communicating.

Faxes

Although used less and less, you may still occasionally be asked to fax something. If you do, use a cover sheet that clearly indicates who the fax is to and from and how many pages you are sending. If some pages do not get properly transmitted, the receiver might not realize they are missing anything if they don't know how many pages you intended to send. Most people today are scanning and emailing or photographing and texting documents rather than faxing or using the good old US Postal Service.

Social Media

Messaging people on Facebook, LinkedIn, Twitter, and so on has also become a popular means of communicating. But one problem is that many people who use those mediums don't regularly check their private messages there. So don't rely on this mode for important communication.

Texting

Because texting is a quick way to get a message to someone, it is great for short, timely messages. Be sure to identify yourself in the message when texting someone for the first time since the recipient may not recognize your phone number. Use few if any abbreviations, and don't rely on spell-check to get it all right.

Technology can be a great tool when used appropriately. However, you'll lose credibility and miss out on many opportunities when it becomes obvious that you haven't learned the rules. Boost your image, your workplace savvy, and your effectiveness by learning and using communication technology in a considerate and responsible way.

Have Business Cards Made

Every nurse needs to have a business card. Why? Because this is how professional people network and exchange contact information. Many nurses are under the mistaken impression that business cards are only for those who own a business. On the contrary, they are simply calling cards used for professional networking. Today, anyone who's anybody has a business card, and every nurse is definitely somebody. Business cards are a professional way of introducing yourself. They create the opportunity to stay in touch with people. People exchange business cards with one another in both social and workplace situations. Besides, having a business card makes you feel important.

If you already have a card from your place of employment, that's fine. However, you may want to have your own cards made with personal contact information on them. This way, people can get in touch with you outside of work and can still reach you if you ever leave your current job. Many of us change jobs more often than we move our place of residence. Of course, you can always write your personal information on the back of your work-related card so that people feel like they're getting special access to you.

If you don't have work-related cards, ask your supervisor if you can get them. Explain they are part of your professional image when you are representing your employer, and that you need them for professional networking both in and outside of your place of employment. Be prepared to sell the idea. It's worth a try. In fact, many nurses who have work-related business cards hand them out to patients and their families in certain circumstances. You have to decide if that's appropriate for you.

In any event, you can have your own cards made easily and inexpensively at any local print shop. And while it is possible to print business cards on your personal computer, it's not recommended because the card stock is flimsy, and the design, layout, and print will not have a truly professional look to it. Your business card makes a statement about you and is part of your professional image. It's a self-marketing tool. Your business card should not appear cheap or homemade. It should convey style and professionalism.

Start with a white card with black lettering for maximum impact. For a professional look, avoid graphics such as flowers. Be sure the type size and font style is easily readable. Ask the printer for recommendations and examples.

Frequently Asked Questions

Q: *What information should be on my personal business card?*

A: Start with your name followed by professional credentials. Include your cell and/or workplace phone number (if you want people to call you at either), and email address (see figure 10-1). You can also include your LinkedIn (LI) URL, if your profile is up to date. Consider including your Twitter handle, but that is optional. Only include your Facebook link if it would add value to your professional persona. Otherwise, leave it off. Of course, people can find it on their own, but there is no need to include it with your professional paperwork. Remember, you won't be giving cards that list your personal information to patients. You'll be using them for professional networking.

Q: *How should I list my credentials after my name on my business card?*

A: This is an age-old question. Some people list their nursing credentials first and their degrees second while others list degrees first and nursing credentials second. Either way is technically correct. However, the American Nurses Credentialing Center (ANCC) recommends that nurses all use a standardized format for listing credentials in the following order:

C: 555-222-4545
B: 555-222-5454

Janet Fredericks, RN, MS

janet@net.net
Linkedin.com/in/janetfredricks
@jfredricks

Figure 10–1. Example of a business card

highest earned degree, licensure, state designations or requirements (e.g., APRN [advanced practice registered nurse], NP [nurse practitioner], CNS [clinical nurse specialist]), national certifications, awards and honors, other recognitions. Here are some examples:

Karen Collins, PhD, RN, FAAN

Robert Allen, MS, RN, CNOR

Katherine Caldwell, BSN, RN

Q: *Should I list my associate degree in nursing (ADN)? If I get a master of science in nursing (MSN), should I drop the bachelor of science in nursing (BSN)?*

A: If you have multiple degrees in nursing, it is most practical to just list the highest degree earned. If you have the same level of degree in both nursing and nonnursing majors such as an MSN and MBA, you may want to list them both, placing the nursing degree first depending on the environment you work in. For example: "Kareen Carol, MSN, MBA, RN." If your highest degree is in a nonnursing major but you also hold a lesser degree in nursing, you may want to list both. For example: "Jake Tapper, MPH, BSN, RN."

Don't get carried away with initials. This is just a calling card, not a bio sketch.

Q: *Should I list things like "CPR certified" or some sort of title or specialty under my name?*

A: It is not necessary or advisable to list credentials like basic life support (BLS) or advanced cardiac life support (ALS) on your business card. It is also not necessary to list something like "psychiatric nurse" or "oncology nurse" under your name, unless you are promoting a consulting practice in that specialty.

Q: *Should I list links to my social media pages on my card?*

A: You can add the professional ones such as LI and Twitter if you wish, but consider adding them to the back of the card so as not to clutter up the front. Example: "Twitter: @DonnaCardilloRN."

Q: *Who needs business cards?*

A: Every nurse and student nurse needs a card whether actively working, retired, between jobs, a full-time student, currently out of the workforce for any reason, and so on. *No one is exempt.*

Q: *How and when would I use a business card?*

A: Once you have business cards, you'll be amazed at all the practical uses and opportunities that exist to exchange contact information. Here are just a few examples:

- Enclose your card when mailing a gift, photo, article, or résumé to someone.
- Exchange cards with colleagues you meet at association meetings, seminars, or conventions so you can stay in touch with them for support and information sharing.
- Present your card when meeting a key media person, author, or industry leader and offer yourself as a resource for future programs and articles.
- Offer your card to someone from a company you always wanted to work for. Ask them to keep you in mind if anything comes up.
- Enclose your business card when sending a greeting card or hand-written note to someone so the person can get in touch with you if they wish.
- Give your card to those you mentor or precept. This way they'll be able to get in touch with you when they need to.
- Provide your card to someone who offers to send you some information.

Use Them!

Once you have business cards made, carry them with you wherever you go. Don't leave them in your office, in your car, at home, or in your hotel room when at a conference. I always have a few business cards with me no matter where I go—and that includes the beach, on vacation, to the beauty parlor, and to social events. You never know whom you'll meet where, and you always want to be prepared.

To add an extra element of style, get a business-card holder to carry in your pocket or purse. This is a small pouch or hinged box. Not only does it make a great presentation, but it keeps your cards from getting dog-eared and dirty. Your card is part of your professional image so keep them clean and up to date. If information changes, get new cards made. Don't cross out the old information and pen in the new info, that's tacky and unprofessional.

Be sure your cards are readily accessible so you don't have to start digging in your purse or wallet to find one. If you're attending a networking event, put a handful of cards in your pocket or other easily accessible place so you can retrieve one with ease. Some people keep their own cards in one pocket and those they collect from others in another.

Q: *Is there a proper way to present my card or ask people for theirs?*

A: Yes! Distribute your cards with discretion. Don't hand them out as if you were dealing out a poker hand. And don't thrust it into someone's hand when you first meet him. Rather, it is appropriate to engage in some conversation with someone before offering your card. Then say something like, "May I give you my card?" or, "I'd like to give you my card." You can add, "Please feel free to call on me if I can help you in any way," "Keep me in your Rolodex and use me as a resource," or, "Perhaps we can talk further after today and share some information." When presenting your card, hand it print side up and facing the receiver so they can read it without turning it.

If someone asks you for your card, and you don't have one with you, don't ever say, "I don't have a card; but if you give me one of yours, I'll write my name and number on the back." Some people find that tacky and offensive—just because you don't have a card doesn't give you the right to use theirs as scrap paper. Rather, write your name and contact information on a piece of paper or offer to send your card to them when you get home. Of course the exception would be if someone offers you their own business card for that express purpose. A better solution is to never be caught without your cards!

When requesting someone else's card, say something like, "May I have your business card?" or, "Do you have a business card?" When accepting someone else's business card, it is polite to look it over for a moment and comment on it. Make note of their name, title, and organization if applicable. You might say, "I see you're located in New York City. Have you been there long?" If it is a workplace card, you might say their title out loud and comment, "What exactly does a director of patient care services do?" You can also say something like, "May I call on you in the future if I have further questions?"

Once you have your business cards, you're ready to move forward.

Firm Up Your Handshaking Technique

If you want to be taken seriously as a nurse, you need to start shaking hands. Handshaking is an important social custom in the western world. Extending your hand to someone is a sign of respect. Proper handshaking will enhance your credibility and put you, along with the entire profession, on a more equal footing with other professions in health care and society in general.

There is a natural and legitimate concern among nurses about the transmission of germs by hand-to-hand contact. However, the opportunity to connect with another person through a respectful form of touching outweighs the potential drawbacks. And good hygiene, including frequent handwashing and the regular use of waterless sanitizer, will minimize any infection control issues.

The handshake is an important part of a first impression. In many situations, people will evaluate you based on whether or not you shake hands and the quality of your handshake. A limp handshake may give the impression that you are an insecure or insincere person, while a firm handshake conveys character and authority, not to mention confidence. I've already mentioned how important the handshake is on a job interview and in networking situations, but there are many other occasions when a handshake should be used as well.

It is particularly important for nurses to shake hands with their patients and patients' families when appropriate. Obviously it would not be appropriate in emergency situations but can be used in many health care settings and situations. As caregivers, nurses have license to have physical contact with others that goes beyond what is usually socially acceptable. Therefore, initially shaking hands with a patient during an introduction is a respectful way of starting the caregiving relationship. It is also a good chance for the patient and nurse to start creating a bond of trust. Likewise, a nurse should shake hands with family members, physicians, and other health care professionals as well as colleagues that you do not see on a regular basis, such as those you see at meetings and conventions.

How to Shake Hands

There are many wrong ways to shake hands but only one right way. (This technique is the same whether shaking hands with a woman or a man.) Approach the person with whom you wish to shake hands. Maintain eye contact with the other person and, when you're about 3 feet away, fully extend your right hand with your thumb pointing up. Engage the other person's hand, making palm-to-palm contact, locking thumb webs. Your fingers should wrap around the other person's hand in a firm grip (don't crush the other person's metacarpals). Then use one or two downward pumps and release the grip, all while maintaining eye contact.

Be sure to smile while you're at it, conveying confidence, warmth, and sincerity. It's a three-pronged approach: a full firm handshake, eye contact, and a smile. A handshake without eye contact is not considered credible. You will encounter some less than desirable handshakes such as the "dead fish" (limp) or "fingertips only." Remain steady with your own firm handshake. You cannot control the other person's handshake; you can only control your own.

If someone is standing and offers to shake your hand, you should stand to shake theirs, whether you are a man or a woman. This promotes a sense of equality in some cases and respect between the parties. Although a handshake will not "equalize" the relationship between an older person and a younger person or a senior person and a junior person in a corporation, it can make a statement that both parties are important in their unique roles. This could be the case with nurses shaking hands with physicians and other health care professionals, for example.

What Not to Do

Just as there is an appropriate way to shake hands, there are some things to avoid:

- Avoid a two-handed shake in which people use their second hand to cover the clasped hands or to enclose the other person's one hand in their two hands. Although often done as a friendly gesture, people can misconstrue this handshake technique as motherly, controlling, or too intimate.

- Do not put your free hand on the other person's shoulder or grip their forearm while shaking hands. By so doing, you step beyond what is socially acceptable and invade their personal space.

- Pause for a moment before pulling your hand out of the shake. Try to be the last person to release the grip. It may seem awkward at first, but you'll get a feel for it with some experience.

- If you pour cologne or perfume into your hands to pat on your face or pulse points, be sure to wash your hands well afterward. You don't want everyone you shake hands with to smell you on their hands for the rest of the day.

When to Shake Hands

Now that you know the proper way to shake hands, when is it appropriate to shake? A handshake should always be used:

- Upon meeting someone for the first time;
- To greet someone you don't see on a regular basis;
- When parting company with those you just met or don't see often;
- At the start and end of an interview, even if you know the person well;
- After a meeting or conversation, to show agreement or solidarity;
- Whenever someone offers their hand to you; and
- When you're welcoming people into your home, your office, or a meeting.

I like to shake hands with members of my audience when I am giving a presentation—either before or after the event. It's a good way to introduce yourself, make attendees feel special, and to make a more personal connection with audience members.

Cultural Differences

Cultural differences exist where handshaking and eye contact are concerned, and it is important for nurses to be aware of some of the differences. While it is common for those from Europe and Australia to shake hands and make direct eye contact, it is much less common in those from Asian countries where less eye contact and a more delicate handshake might be the preferred norm. This does not mean that you must adapt your handshake depending on someone's country of origin. It simply means that you should be aware that differences exist so that you do not misin-terpret someone else's habits or behaviors.

Also, some men of orthodox Jewish and Muslim faiths are not permitted to have physical contact with a woman other than a close family member. So how do you know who to extend your hand to and who not to? In some cases, you can identify a man of orthodox Jewish faith by his distinctive dress. With that exception, it is better to extend your hand in most situations as a gesture of good will. If the other person cannot shake hands for religious reasons, they will usually graciously state, "My culture does not permit me to shake hands," or something similar. In that case you would simply drop your hand back to your side and nod a greeting. There is no reason for embarrassment or feelings of being slighted.

People with Disabilities

Just because someone has a disability, it doesn't mean you should bypass the traditional handshake. This convention is important with people who are disabled and who are often marginalized or treated differently. As nurses, we have a responsibility to be role models for greetings and behaviors that are respectful and appropriate for all people, especially those with a physical or mental disability.

If someone is visually impaired, you might ask, "May I shake your hand?" and then bring your hand to meet theirs. If someone has a missing or nonfunctioning right hand or limb, offer your left hand to shake. Likewise, if someone offers the left hand first for whatever reason, meet it with your left. If someone has limited use of both limbs, extend your right hand anyway close to their right hand. People with a limitation will usually make an effort to meet your hand in some capacity. If shaking isn't possible, a nod of the head or a light touch on the hand is appropriate to acknowledge the person.

Troubleshooting

Even with the best of intentions, there are often obstacles and stumbling blocks to something as seemingly simple as a handshake. They might include:

- **Being unable to shake hands.** If, for example, you've had recent hand surgery or have severe arthritis, you might politely say something like, "Forgive me for not shaking your hand, but I recently had hand surgery."
- **Having cold hands or sweaty palms.** Shake anyway. The receiver is generally much less aware of the state of your hand than you are.

Don't apologize for your cold or sweaty hands and draw attention to them. Of course, if you know beforehand that you will be greeting someone and shaking hands, you can prepare. If your hands are cold, rub them together when no one is looking. If you have sweaty palms, keep a handkerchief in your pocket and use it discreetly, if possible, just before shaking to dry off your hand. If that's not feasible, shake hands anyway. The act of shaking hands is more important than the fact that your hand is sweaty or cold. If you refuse to shake, people may assume that you are unfriendly or do not respect them.

- *Refusing to shake someone's extended hand is insulting unless you offer an acceptable reason, such as religious proscription or physical limitation.*

- **Getting brushed off.** If you extend your hand to someone to shake, and they do not respond, simply drop your hand to your side and carry on. Who knows what their motivation is. Just don't take it personally.

- **Having your hands full (literally).** If you're holding something in your right hand when someone approaches you to shake hands, put whatever it is down or shift it to your left hand. At networking and social events, carry a drink in your left hand so you are prepared to shake hands. You can also extend your left hand, if necessary, in a pinch.

- **Proper handshaking conveys confidence, trust, and openness.** If you already have a good, firm handshake and use it regularly, you're ahead of the game. If not, start practicing to perfect your grip and begin using your newly acquired skill.

Brush Up on Your Conversational Skills

"Don't talk to strangers" is the warning we grew up with. So it's natural to feel uncomfortable striking up a conversation with people you don't know. Most of us are reluctant to walk up to strangers and introduce ourselves. But if you work to overcome this, you will have the social advantage. Here are some strategies that work.

If you find yourself at an event with no one to talk to, look for someone who also appears to be alone rather than trying to break into a group discussion. If you use your observational skills, you'll get a sense of who is open to talking versus those who seem to want to be alone. If you approach someone who won't make eye contact or smile and who seems distracted or disinterested, just move on. You might also approach the food table, if there is one, and say to someone there, "This looks good. Do they always put out this kind of spread?"

If you're feeling out of the loop and not up on what's happening in the world, read a weekly news magazine before going out. These publications usually provide a good overview of world events, domestic news, pop culture, and the latest book, movie, and music releases.

Be observant and find something to compliment, like a piece of jewelry, a tie, or article of clothing. Most of us appreciate a sincere compliment, and often there's a story associated with the item like a great vacation or holiday. Now you've started a light conversation.

I've had interesting conversation with people I've encountered on airplanes and in the hair salon by commenting on a book they were reading or carrying. You might say, "I noticed you are reading Stephen King's latest book, and I was thinking of buying it. Are you enjoying it?" There are opportunities to network virtually everywhere.

If you're attending a seminar or workshop, you might ask fellow attendees on a break, "How do you like the program so far?" or, "Where did you travel from today?" These are easily answered icebreakers that invite further conversation. They open the door for you to introduce yourself and extend your hand for a handshake. Many people will welcome your initiative with a sigh of relief for getting the ball rolling. Warming up with an icebreaker or two makes self-introduction much less intimidating.

How do you keep the ball rolling once you get it going? It's always a good idea to stay focused on the other person by showing interest in them and what they do. It's said that everyone's favorite subject to talk about is him- or herself. Ask a few simple yes-or-no or open-ended questions such as, "Are you a member of this association? For how long? What do like about it?" Be sure to offer like information about yourself, too, without monopolizing the conversation. Networking is a reciprocal, give-and-take relationship. It's only through self-disclosure that you'll reap the maximum benefit.

Avoid the "hot" topics like politics, religion, and anything you're passionate about where you can't tolerate another opinion. Safe topics of conversation are the weather, certain current events, sports and entertainment, and industry issues. If you're sitting at a table with others, you might say, "Did anyone see the news story about [fill in the blank]?" or, "Has anyone seen the movie [fill in the blank]?" Choose a topic in which you're interested or have some expertise. With some practice, you will overcome your shyness and fear of talking to people.

Finding a Mentor

There is an abundance of material available on how to be a good mentor, but very little is written on how to find one. How can you find the right person to advise, guide, and coach you? And how do you approach that person once you do find them? Consider the following points.

Getting Started

Think about what you want to accomplish before contacting a potential mentor. Are you looking to advance in your current place of employment, succeed in a new job, or do you simply want to be better in your chosen specialty? A mentor can be helpful in a variety of situations and in various phases of your career. However, experienced nurses who want to make the move to the next level or make a change within their career often benefit most from being mentored.

What to Look For

When considering a potential mentor, look for someone whom you admire and respect. It is also important to find someone who is experienced and successful in their profession or specialty, not to mention well connected. Likewise, it is advantageous to seek out someone who seems approachable and friendly and who is passionate and enthusiastic about their work; in other words, someone you would feel comfortable with.

Where to Look

Someone who is self-employed or who works for a different employer than you do is more likely to be your mentor. But don't overlook someone who works with you. Consider a current or former instructor or someone who holds a position you aspire to as a mentor, even if they are retired.

Some professional associations have mentoring programs that match experienced colleagues with up-and-coming members.

How to Initiate the Relationship

Make a list of all the people you know who fit the preceding descriptions. Has any one of them shown an interest in you and your career? Has anyone been particularly helpful? Possibly you're surrounded by potential mentors, people giving you advice and guidance. You need to take the lead and see if any of them are willing to develop a more formal relationship.

In some cases, it's better to let the relationship develop naturally. Perhaps you've been getting occasional advice from a former supervisor or instructor. Maybe there is someone you simply know or admire. Contact that person and let them know how much you respect them and value their opinion and that you aspire to be more like them. Ask if you could meet with them for 20–30 minutes to learn more about them. You should then begin to develop a sense of the person's comfort with—and the potential for—a more formal relationship with you.

You may need or want to approach someone who does not know you. In this case, you might initially send a letter of introduction expressing your interest in speaking with that person, noting that you will call them as follow-up. Express your interest in that person and your value of their experience. But don't mention the possibility of mentoring in the letter. Once you have met and established a relationship, then you can ask if they would be willing to mentor you to work toward achieving your career goals.

Keep in mind that some people simply do not have the time or energy to be a mentor, so don't take it personally if that is the response you get. Maintain a relationship with that person anyway and look for another prospective mentor.

How to Be a Good Protégé

All relationships are reciprocative; both parties must benefit. Your mentor will benefit from your feedback regarding their advice, both good and bad. Always keep your mentor posted on your progress. Support your mentor in several ways, such as nominating them for awards. Always be ready to show your appreciation by referring potential clients or by passing on information and resources that may be of interest to them, if appropriate.

Additional Considerations

Can your boss be your mentor? It's possible but not ideal. The need to discuss sometimes sensitive workplace issues and on-the-job politics and competition favors a mentor to whom you don't report. Also, you needn't be of the same gender or in the same specialty as your mentor.

All relationships change over time, so you are likely to have several mentors over the course of your career. Don't take the hard road and do things on your own. Most successful people were guided and supported by mentors. Seek these people out for success.

Put Yourself First

The critical flaw in caregiving is that care for the caregiver often has the lowest priority. Airline passengers are cautioned, in an emergency, that they should put their oxygen masks on first before helping others. That is because if they become incapacitated, then they are of no use to themselves or others. Nurses are professional caregivers. We can see firsthand the effects of having little time and energy for ourselves: stress, illness, short tempers, loss of focus and perspective, poor judgment, and errors. When you are overtaxed, things start to go wrong. It's impossible to avoid stress, but you can fight its effects.

Find Respite in Your Day

The more extended your efforts become, the less effective you may be, and the more likely you may be to make mistakes. How many nurses regularly skip breaks and meals? It is imperative to pause for recovery and renewal, even if for a few minutes at a time. Shift your focus to other matters by stepping outside, sitting in a chapel or meditation room, or taking a few deep breaths in another quiet spot.

Rediscover Yourself

A frantic pace in everyday life can sweep away our sense of self. When I ask nurses what they enjoy doing, some cannot answer the question because it's been so long since they did anything for fun. They have become so unaccustomed to having free time with activities of their own.

Try journaling, creating self-portrait collages (cutting out words, images, and symbols from magazines that you identify with and pasting them on poster board), and listening to music from your youth to help regain a sense of self. Spend time with a hobby, take up an artistic pursuit, or commune with nature. Balance the demands of our profession by creating a full, satisfying life outside of work.

Get Physical

The Greek philosopher Aristotle described humans as psychosomatic, or mind–body entities. For either to function well, both mind and body need to be healthy; they are the two inseparable parts of the whole person. Exercise lowers stress, improves health, controls weight, elevates mood, and more. Nurses know this but ignore it too often. It is as if they think they're exempt from the advice they give their patients. And don't think being busy all day equates exercise; it doesn't by a long shot.

A daily walking routine is a good way to start, combining exercise with time to be alone with your thoughts. Some of us will find that a health club or fitness center suits us better. Exercise alone or get a workout buddy or two. You'll find yourselves sharing and venting as you walk, jog, or stretch together. Dancing, cycling, and swimming are great pursuits to invigorate the body, clear the mind, and work off the day's travails.

Use Relaxation Techniques
Think of yourself as a reservoir of mental and physical energy that needs to be refilled before running dry. Meditation, yoga, stretching, and deep breathing will refill the reservoir and rejuvenate the spirit. They can be done virtually anywhere. They are widely practiced today, and loads of books and articles on all three topics have been written to guide you in proper techniques. Don't overlook the benefits of massage, Reiki, and acupressure. These are necessities, not luxuries, for easing tension and tight muscles, and for realigning physical, mental and spiritual energy. Ask for gift certificates to salons and spas for birthdays and holidays. Don't wait; tend to yourself now because relaxation is routine maintenance for the mind, body, and spirit.

Care for the caregiver is top priority to ensure you can take care of everyone else with the focus, stamina, and enthusiasm they deserve.

Stop Apologizing All the Time
When you say you're sorry all the time, it sounds as if you're taking the blame for everything that happens. It's annoying to many people, and it makes you seem like a self-appointed scapegoat. Don't say "I'm sorry" unless you've done something for which you truly need to apologize.

Learn to Take a Compliment
When complimented on a job well done, many managers, project leaders and association executives I've known respond, "Oh, I didn't do anything. It was the team that did all the work." A more appropriate response would be to say, "Thank you. I had a great team to work with on this." Accepting a genuine compliment is not a sign of conceit. It's simply a gracious way

of appreciating someone's acknowledgment of something you did. How many times has someone said to you, "Thanks for what you did for me," and you responded, "It was nothing," or "Don't mention it," thereby minimizing your actions? A more assertive reply would be "It was my pleasure," or "I'm happy I was able to help." This type of response is important because when you deflect a compliment, you're basically saying, "My actions were meaningless or minimal and unworthy of acknowledgement."

Don't Be Self-Deprecating

While modesty is an admirable trait, taking it to an extreme is counterproductive. Self-deprecation belittles you, working from the inside to sabotage your work and value. I once attended an awards ceremony sponsored by a local nursing organization. Several RNs were being honored for outstanding work in the field. One nurse walked up to the podium after being introduced and said, "I don't deserve this award." In her well-meaning attempt to not appear boastful, she negated the contributions of all nurses. Her comments were unnecessary and inappropriate. She simply might have said, "I'm honored and humbled by this recognition. I accept this award on behalf of all my fellow nurses who do such outstanding work every day and often remain in the shadows."

Act Confident Even If You Don't Feel Confident

Force yourself to make good eye contact with people and use a steady, audible voice when speaking. Stand or sit erect with your head upright and straight on your shoulders, not tilted to the side or bent forward. Act like you have a right to be there, even if you don't yet feel that way. If someone attempts to interrupt you while you're talking, keep talking until you are done and raise the volume of your voice if necessary to be heard. If you stop talking midstream in an effort to be "polite," you are making a statement that they have more of a right to speak than you do.

Being assertive is not about being combative or aggressive. It's about firmly holding a belief that you're someone who matters. Acting in a more assertive manner actually will make you feel more assertive and lead to increased confidence. Just as important, it will help you get noticed and listened to and start to garner the respect you and your profession deserve. Take some small steps in the right direction today.

Create a Professional Image

Last but certainly not least is the subject of appearance and image. While we already discussed the importance of appearance on a job interview, your appearance and overall image post-hire will be a major factor in your future success—or lack of it. Having a license, credentials, and experience are simply not enough to convey professionalism and character. You have to look the part of a professional nurse as well as be the part. You have to inspire confidence in others. Simply put, you have to develop a professional image, both online and in-person, to match the professional person you are.

Whether you work in a hospital, office, corporate setting, or in the field, your appearance matters. Your clothing, your grooming, and your accessories make a loud statement about who you are and what you stand for. You represent your entire profession and other professional nurses whenever you interact with others, so keep that in mind.

First impressions and overall image impact our professional and personal lives every day in every situation. Nonverbal communication accounts for more than half of the message you send out when interacting with people. Like it or not, people judge us based on our appearance just as we do with others.

Whether you wear scrubs, uniforms, business casual clothes, or business suits, you should always be conservatively and meticulously attired and groomed in workplace and professional settings. In the movie *Working Girl* (1988), actor Melanie Griffith, while trying to rise above her dead-end job, realizes that she has to change her image if she wants to get ahead. She utters the line, "If you want to be taken seriously, you need serious hair." You also need "serious" clothes and "serious" accessories.

Conclusion

In summary, whether happy in your current position, unemployed, or looking to make a change, it is vital to always be moving forward in your career. To make positive changes and create momentum in your professional life, you don't have to take a big leap of faith or make radical changes. Rather, you can start making small changes today, putting one foot in front of the other and moving forward in a positive direction. Move forward in faith and enjoy the journey!

I want to hear from you after you've finished reading this book. Please write to me and let me know how you used the information and the strategies provided. Tell me about your career, lessons you've learned, rewards, challenges, and so on. I look forward to hearing from you!

Donna Cardillo, RN, MA, CSP
PO Box 15
Sea Girt, NJ 08750
Donna@DonnaCardillo.com

Find Donna on Facebook, LinkedIn, Twitter, Instagram, and Pinterest.

Resources

References

Brown, H. J., Jr. (1996). *A Hero in Every Heart: Champions from All Walks of Life Share Powerful Messages to Inspire the Hero in Each of Us.* Nashville, TN: T. Nelson.

Clinical Nurse Leader Association. (2017). "What is a CNL?" www.cnlassociation.org/about/what-is-a-cnl.

Leonard, M., & Miller, E. (2012). *Nursing Case Management: Review and Resource Manual.* 4th ed. Silver Spring, MD: American Nurses Credentialing Center.

Recommended Reading

Bolles, R. *What Color Is Your Parachute?: A Practical Manual for Job-Hunters and Career-Changers.* Berkeley, CA: Ten Speed Press, 2018.

Cardillo, D. *A Daybook for Beginning Nurses.* Indianapolis, IN: Sigma Theta Tau International, 2010.

Cardillo, D. *Falling Together: How to Find Balance, Joy, and Meaningful Change When Your Life Seems to Be Falling Apart.* Berkley, CA: She Writes Press, 2016.

Cardillo, D. *Your First Year as a Nurse: Making the Transition from Total Novice to Successful Professional.* 2nd ed. New York, NY: Three Rivers Press, 2010.

Carlson, K. *Savvy Networking for Nurses: Getting Connected (and Staying Connected) in the 21st Century.* Santa Fe, NM; Author, 2015.

Maheady, D. C. *Leave No Nurse Behind: Nurses Working with disAbilities.* Lincoln, NB: iUniverse, Inc., 2006.

Pagana, K. *The Nurse's Etiquette Advantage: How Professional Etiquette Can Advance Your Nursing Career.* 2nd ed. Indianapolis, IN: Sigma Theta Tau International, 2015.

Sullivan, E. J. *Becoming Influential: A Guide for Nurses.* 2nd ed. London: Pearson, 2012.

Wilson, B. *The Nerdy Nurse's Guide to Technology.* Indianapolis, IN: Sigma Theta Tau International, 2014.

National Nursing Organizations

American Nurses Association
www.nursingworld.org

National Association of Licensed Practical Nurses
nalpn.org

National League for Nursing (NLN)
www.nln.org

National Student Nurses Association
www.nsna.org

Specialty Nursing Associations*

American Academy of Medical Esthetic Professionals (formerly Association of Medical Esthetic Nurses)
www.aamep.org

Academy of Medical Surgical Nurses
www.amsn.org

Air & Surface Transport Nurses Association
www.astna.org

American Academy of Ambulatory Care Nursing
www.aaacn.org

American Assisted Living Nurses Association
www.alnursing.org

American Association of Critical-Care Nurses
www.aacn.org

American Association of Diabetes Educators
www.diabeteseducator.org

American Association of Heart Failure Nurses
www.aahfn.org

American Association of Legal Nurse Consultants
www.aalnc.org

American Association of Managed Care Nurses
www.aamcn.org

American Association of Moderate Sedation Nurses
www.aamsn.org

American Association of Neuroscience Nurses
www.aann.org

American Association of Nurse Assessment Coordination
www.aanac.org

American Association of Nurse Attorneys
www.taana.org

American Association of Nurse Life Care Planners
www.aanlcp.org

American Association of Occupational Health Nurses
www.aaohn.org

American Association of Spinal Cord Injury Nurses
www.aascin.org

American Cannabis Nurses Association
www.cannabisnurses.org

American Holistic Nurses Association
www.ahna.org

American Nephrology Nurses Association
www.annanurse.org

American Psychiatric Nurses Association
www.apna.org

American Public Health Association
www.apha.org

American Nursing Informatics Association
www.ania.org

American Society of Ophthalmic Registered Nurses
www.asorn.org

American Society of Pain Management Nursing
www.aspmn.org

American Society of PeriAnesthesia Nurses
www.aspan.org

American Society of Plastic and Aesthetic Nurses
www.aspsn.org

Association for Nursing Professional Development (formerly National Nursing Staff Development Organization)
www.anpd.org

Association of Camp Nursing
www.acn.org

Association of Child Neurology Nurses
www.childneurologysociety.org/acnn

Association of Clinical Documentation Improvement Specialists
www.acdis.org

Association of Community Health Nursing Educators
www.achne.org

American Organization of Nurse Executives
www.aone.org

Association of Nurses in AIDS Care
www.nursesinaidscare.org

Association of Pediatric Hematology/
Oncology Nurses
www.aphon.org

Association of periOperative Registered
Nurses
www.aorn.org

Association for Professionals in Infection
Control and Epidemiology
www.apic.org

Association for Radiologic & Imaging
Nursing
www.arinursing.org

Association of Rehabilitation Nurses
www.rehabnurse.org

Association of Women's Health, Obstetric
and Neonatal Nurses
www.awhonn.org

Baromedical Nurses Association
www.hyperbaricnurses.org

Case Management Society of America
www.cmsa.org

Clinical Nurse Leader Association
www.cnlassociation.org

Dermatology Nurses' Association
www.dnanurse.org

Developmental Disabilities Nurses
Association
www.ddna.org

Emergency Nurses Association
www.ena.org

Endocrine Nurses Society
www.endo-nurses.org

Home Healthcare Nurses Association
www.hhna.org

Hospice & Palliative Nurses Association
www.hpna.org

Infusion Nurses Society
www.ins1.org

International Association of Forensic
Nurses
www.forensicnurses.org

International Organization of Multiple
Sclerosis Nurses
www.iomsn.org

International Nurses Society on
Addictions
www.intnsa.org

International Society of Nurses in Cancer
Care
www.isncc.org

International Transplant Nurses Society
www.itns.org

National Association of Directors of
Nursing Administration in Long Term
Care
www.nadona.org

National Association of Neonatal Nurses
www.nann.org

National Association of Nurse Massage
Therapists
www.nanmt.org

National Association of Orthopaedic
Nurses
www.orthonurse.org

National Association of School Nurses
www.nasn.org

National Association of School Nurses for
the Deaf
www.nasnd.net

National Association of State School
Nurse Consultants
www.schoolnurseconsultants.org

National Gerontological Nursing
Association
www.aginginmotion.org

National Nurses in Business Association
www.nnbanow.com

Nurses Organization of Veterans Affairs
www.vanurse.org

Oncology Nursing Society
www.ons.org

Pediatric Endocrinology Nursing Society
www.pens.org

Respiratory Nursing Society
www.respiratorynursingsociety.org

Rheumatology Nurses Society
www.rnsnurse.org

Society of Gastroenterology Nurses and
Associates
www.sgna.org

Society of Gynecological Nurse Oncologists
www.sgno.org

Society of Otorhinolaryngology and Head-Neck Nurses
www.sohnnurse.com

Society of Pediatric Nurses
www.pedsnurses.org

Society of Trauma Nurses
www.traumanurses.org

Society of Urological Nurses and Associates
www.suna.org

Society for Vascular Nursing
www.svnnet.org

Space Nursing Society
www.spacenursingsociety.org

Transcultural Nursing Society
www.tcns.org

Wound Ostomy and Continence Nurses Society
www.wocn.org

Advanced Practice Nursing Associations*

Advanced Practitioner Society for Hematology and Oncology
www.apsho.org

American Academy of Emergency Nurse Practitioners
www.aaenp-natl.org

American Association of Nurse Anesthetists
www.aana.com

American Association of Nurse Practitioners
www.aanp.org

American College of Nurse-Midwives
www.midwife.org

Doctors of Nursing Practice
www.doctorsofnursingpractice.org

Gerontological Advanced Practice Nurses Association
www.gapna.org

International Council of Nurse Practitioners
www.icn-apnetwork.org

National Academy of Dermatology Nurse Practitioners
www.nadnp.net

National Association of Clinical Nurse Specialists
www.nacns.org

National Organization of Nurse Practitioner Faculties
www.nonpf.org

National Association of Pediatric Nurse Practitioners
www.napnap.org

Nurse Practitioners in Women's Health
www.npwh.org

ANA State Nurses Associations

Alabama State Nurses Association
www.alabamanurses.org

Arizona Nurses Association
www.aznurse.org

Arkansas Nurses Association
www.arna.org

ANA California
www.anacalifornia.org

Colorado Nurses Association
www.coloradonurses.org

Connecticut Nurses Association
www.ctnurses.org

Delaware Nurses Association
www.denurses.org

Florida Nurses Association
www.floridanurse.org

Georgia Nurses Association
www.georgianurses.org

Guam Nurses Association
www.guamnursesassociation.org

ANA Idaho
www.idahonurses.org

ANA Illinois
www.ana-illinois.org

Indiana State Nurses Association
www.indiananurses.org

Iowa Nurses Association
www.iowanurses.org

Kansas State Nurses Association
www.ksnurses.com

ANA Kentucky
www.kentucky-nurses.org

Louisiana State Nurses Association
www.lsna.org

ANA Maine
www.anamaine.org

Maryland Nurses Association
www.marylandrn.org

ANA Massachusetts
www.anamass.org

ANA Michigan
www.ana-michigan.org

Minnesota Nurses Association
www.mnorn.org

Mississippi Nurses Association
www.msnurses.org

Missouri Nurses Association
www.missourinurses.org

Montana Nurses Association
www.mtnurses.org

Nebraska Nurses Association
www.NebraskaNurses.org

Nevada Nurses Association
www.nvnurses.org

New Hampshire Nurses Association
www.NHnurses.org

New Jersey State Nurses Association
www.njsna.org

New Mexico Nurses Association
www.nmna.org

ANA New York
www.ANA-NewYork.org

North Carolina Nurses Association
www.ncnurses.org

North Dakota Nurses Association
www.ndna.org

Ohio Nurses Association
www.ohnurses.org

Oklahoma Nurses Association
www.oklahomanurses.org

Oregon Nurses Association
www.oregonrn.org

Pennsylvania State Nurses Association
www.psna.org

ANA Rhode Island
www.risna.org

South Carolina Nurses Association
www.scnurses.org

South Dakota Nurses Association
www.sdnursesassociation.org

Tennessee Nurses Association
www.tnaonline.org

Texas Nurses Association
www.texasnurses.org

Utah Nurses Association
www.utnurse.org

ANA Vermont
www.ana-vermont.org

Virgin Islands State Nurses Association
www.visnaus.org

Virginia Nurses Association
www.virginianurses.com

Washington State Nurses Association
www.wsna.org

West Virginia Nurses Association
www.wvnurses.org

Wisconsin Nurses Association
www.wisconsinnurses.org

Wyoming Nurses Association
www.wyonurse.org

Additional State Nurses Association

Alaska Nurses Association
www.aknurse.org

California Nurses Association
www.nationalnursesunited.org/
california-nurses-association

District of Columbia Nurses Association
(subset of National Nursed United)
www.dcna.org

Hawaii Nurses Association
www.hawaiinurses.org

Illinois Nurses Association
www.illinoisnurses.com

Maine State Nurses Association (subset of
National Nurses United)
www.nationalnursesunited.org/nnoc/
maine

Massachusetts State Nursing Association
www.massnurses.org

Michigan Nurses Association
www.minurses.org

New York State Nurses Association
www.nysna.org

Military Nurse Associations
Army Nurse Corps Association
www.e-anca.org

Navy Nurse Corps Association
www.nnca.org

Society of Air Force Nurses, Inc.
www.safn.org

Special Interest Groups*

American Assembly for Men in Nursing
www.aamn.org

Asian American / Pacific Islander Nurses
Association
www.aapina.org

National Alaska Native American Indian
Nurses Association
www.nanainanurses.org

National American Arab Nurses
Association
www.n-aana.org

National Association of Hispanic Nurses
nahnnet.org

National Association of Indian Nurses in
America
www.nainausa.com

National Association of Nigerian Nurses
in North America
www.nannna.org

National Black Nurses Association
www.nbna.org

Nurses Christian Fellowship
www.ncf-jcn.org

Orthodox Jewish Nurses Association
www.ojna.org

Philippine Nurses Association of America
www.mypnaa.org

International Nursing Associations

International Council of Nurses
www.icn.ch

Sigma (Formerly Sigma Theta Tau
International)
www.nursingsociety.org

* Many individual states have additional specialty and special interest groups. Check
with your ANA state association for additional local resources.

Index

About the Author

Donna Wilk Cardillo, RN, MA, CSP (certified speaking professional) is known as the Inspiration Nurse, the Career Guru for Nurses, and the Nurse Whisperer. She travels the world helping nurses to find happiness in their careers and to reach their full potential. She is fiercely passionate about nursing and about life in general.

Donna was the original Dear Donna columnist at Nurse.com and the former health care careers expert at Monster.com. Donna is an expert blogger at DoctorOz.com.

Donna has authored several other books: *Falling Together: How to Find Balance, Joy, and Meaningful Change When Your Life Seems to be Falling Apart; Your First Year as a Nurse: Making the Transition from Total Novice to Successful Professional; A Daybook for Beginning Nurses.* She is creator of the *Career Alternatives for Nurses* seminar and home study program.

Donna has received numerous awards and recognitions, but she is most proud of being named a Diva in Nursing by the Institute for Nursing in New Jersey for outstanding achievements and excellence in practice.

Donna is a lifelong New Jersey resident—an original Jersey girl. She lives "down the shore" in Sea Girt, NJ, with her husband Joe.